Positive Answers

Final Report of
The Wagner Development Group

LONDON: HMSO

Contents

CHAPTER ONE

Introduction

Gillian Wagner OBE

The natural response to a sufficiently strong measure of public concern is to set up a review or to have an inquiry and in due course a series of recommendations are published, amid a certain amount of publicity. Thought is seldom given as to how the recommendations are to be implemented unless the committee concerned has the blessing of the Department of Health, as was the case for both the Seebohm and Griffiths Reports. There are no mechanisms routinely in place to ensure that recommendations made by reviews are properly considered.

The Wagner Development Group was set up after the publication of 'A Positive Choice'[1] specifically to ensure that the Review into Residential Care was fully considered, that conscious decisions were made about its recommendations, priorities set and programmes of work identified. 'Positive Answers' brings together the work of the Wagner Development Group. The composition of the Group reflected the mixed economy of welfare within which the Review recommendations had to be implemented and included the statutory, voluntary and private sectors, employers and trade unions, health, housing, central and local government. Generously funded by foundations and trusts, the Group had the great advantage of being truly independent. It is to be hoped that the Wagner Development Group will provide a model for monitoring progress and pushing forward implementation where key recommendations have not been taken up. The WDG was based at the National Institute for Social Work, and a particular debt of gratitude is owed to the Director, Daphne Statham, to whose support and encouragement the WDG owes much. It is greatly to be hoped that the example of the WDG will encourage others to take matters forward in a similar manner when necessary.

The Wagner Report had already broken new ground in that it had commissioned research reviews, published in 1987 under the title 'The Research Reviewed', which gave the Committee the necessary background and influenced its thinking. As Professor Roy Parker said in his introductory chapter, 'No informed conclusion about the future of residential care can be reached without some understanding and appreciation of those forces which have shaped its history.' 'Positive Answers' is the third volume in the series, and provides an account of the work that has been done since the Wagner Report was published five years ago, as well as looking to the future and underlining the continuing need for the residential sector to highlight good practice; to push for change where this is lacking; to urge that the needs of users, staff, relatives and carers are given the priority they have a right to expect.

Terry Philpot, in the his 'Overview', looks at the changes that have taken place in the five years since the Committee reported and assesses how the Report's findings and the work of the Wagner Development Group have been affected by the developments that have taken place. It is a valuable contribution, setting the work of the Review in a wider perspective and enabling its influence to be assessed in the context of changing legislation and the later reports on the shortcomings of residential care, particularly in the child care field. We are not at the end of the long dark tunnel down which residential care has journeyed for so long and where glimpses of light are rare, he writes, 'but Wagner has created enough ways through which that light may find a way'. A fair, if sombre, tribute. There is no doubt that recommendations concerning aspects of quality in residential care have progressed, and if Wagner created one of the apertures through which that particular ray of light could penetrate it is a significant gain.

One of the fundamental philosophical concepts underlying the Wagner Report was the importance it gave to ensuring that the needs and wishes of the users should be at the very heart of the service. The question of rights versus responsibilities is a minefield which few have dared to explore in depth and we are grateful to David Lane, in his chapter on 'Rights, Responsibilities, Relationships and Regulations,' for tackling the confusions that surround the subject. His bold and imaginative chapter explores the complexities of the issue of residents' rights and points to the urgency for the need that this issue be analysed and discussed in every training qualifying course, in every agency, in every home. The reason is simple: 'The common features of every major scandal in residential care are the abuse of power by staff and the vulnerability of the residents'.

The work of the Sub-Groups of the Wagner Development Committee forms the core of 'Positive Answers'. We are deeply grateful to the small but dedicated group of people, determined that the issues concerning residential care should neither be ignored nor forgotten except when scandals bring headline news, who gave up so much time and energy to produce their reports. I pay tribute to them all, in particular their chairs, Ian Baillie, Dick Clough, Adele Jones, Barbara Kahan, David Lane, George Mabon, Barbara Meredith, Marissa Micallef and Jane Minter. The report, 'Charter for Children and Young People Living in Groups', chaired by Barbara Kahan will be published separately. The unfailing efficiency of Wendy Beecher, the WDG's secretary and co-editor with Daphne Statham of the 'Wagner Development Group News Bulletin', has greatly contributed to the success of the WDG. Without the generous support of the Tudor Trust, the Baring Foundation and the Carnegie (UK) Trust there would have been no WDG in the first place, and we are grateful to the Department of Health for their benevolent involvement, genuine support and encouragement.

'Positive Answers' not only brings together the work of the Sub-Groups of the WDG, but it also provides a link with the work of the Caring in Homes Initiative, set up in 1989 as a three year programme of developmental work by the Department of Health. The Caring in Homes Initiative makes a major contribution to the positive answers that have flowed from the Wagner Review recommendations. The common concern of both bodies has been to ensure that the quality of life for people living in residential establishments might be improved and assured. For only then will the fundamental change in the public perception of the residential sector, which 'A Positive Choice' sought to promote, become a reality.

The idea that the needs of the users must be given primacy no longer seems surprising; it is an accepted fact, only sadly it is still far from being a reality. But the needs of carers have scarcely begun to be addressed and the part relatives can play has still to impinge in any significant way in the planning and management of residential care. Users, their relatives, and carers are all part of the community and their views and needs have to be taken into account in this new world of assessment and contracting out. It was not something that we considered in 1988, but looking forward into the future these are some of the issues that need to be kept alive.

In conclusion it needs to be stressed that 'Positive Answers' represents a first attempt at answering many of the issues that remain to be addressed now that residential care is accepted as central to the agenda of welfare provision. From security of tenure to training, from residents' rights to the needs of ethnic minorities, there are still a large number of issues that need discussion and action in some cases leading to legislative changes. In handing over the baton, so to speak, the Wagner Development Group very much hopes that a successor body will be set up to take forward the case for promoting the cause of the most vulnerable members of society, be they users of services, their relatives or carers as well as considering the needs of the staff who manage the establishments and care for the residents.

Ensuring the Quality of Residential Services—
A New Agenda

'A Positive Choice' listed ten recommendations to ensure the quality of residential care. The response to each of these original recommendations is fully discussed in Chapter Four. But it seems appropriate at this juncture, in the light of 'Positive Answers', reviewed here, to set forth a revised list, as guidance for future action.

1. A body to take over from the Wagner Development Group to continue to keep the needs of the residential care sector under review.

2. Security of tenure—more work needs to be done to enhance residents' rights.

3. Consideration to be given to a unified registration and inspection system for residential and nursing homes.

4. Training issues need to be addressed.

5. Complaints procedures in statutory, voluntary and private sectors need to be more accessible to residents.

6. The special needs of people from ethnic minorities need to be given particular attention as a matter of urgency.

7. Development of mechanisms to enable discussion of difficult areas about restraint and control with relatives before a crisis develops.

8. Comprehensive information should be readily accessible about the range of services available.

9. Effort should be put into promoting relationships between residential establishments and relatives to enable them to play as full a part as they can.

10. Every means available should be used to contact informal carers to find out what services they need.

It will be interesting, five years hence, to monitor progress achieved.

Note

1. Independent Review into Residential Care (Wagner Committee), *Residential Care: A Positive Choice*, HMSO, 1988.

Wagner Development Group
Current Membership November 1992

Ian Baillie
Director of Social Work, Church of Scotland Board of Social Responsibility

Charlie Barker
British Association of Social Workers

Chris Beddoe
Consultant, Chris Beddoe & Associates

Jefferson Boyce
Association of Black Social Workers and Allied Professionals

Stephen Campbell
Association of County Councils

Richard Clough
Social Care Association

John Findlay
National Association of Local Government Officers

Ian Gilmour
Association of Directors of Social Work/Convention of Scottish
Local Authorities

Lionel Harrison
Observer, Department of Health

Stephen Hey
British Federation of Care Home Proprietors

Simon Hiller
Observer, Department of Health

Linda Hunt
Observer, Social Work Services Group, Scottish Office

Barbara Kahan
Child Care Open Learning Project

David Lane
Association of Directors of Social Services

Margaret Lilwall
National Care Homes Association

George Mabon
United Care Associations

Sheila Mann
Consultant, Psychiatry of Old Age, Homerton Hospital

Paul Martin
Observer, Social Services Inspectorate, Northern Ireland

Barbara Meredith
National Council for Voluntary Organisations

Marisa Micallef
National Council for Voluntary Organisations

John Mooney
Observer, Social Services Inspectorate, Welsh Office

Chris Payne
National Institute for Social Work

Daphne Statham
National Institute for Social Work

Sarah Veale
Trades Union Congress

Lady Wagner
Chairman (June 1990—November 1992)

Peter Westland
Association of Metropolitan Authorities

Mary Winner
Central Council for Education and Training in Social Work

Penny Youll
Caring in Homes Initiative, Brunel University

Past Members

Hugh Barr
Central Council for Education and Training in Social Work

Deidre Dowie
Convention of Scottish Local Authorities

Ray Earwicker
Trades Union Congress

Adrienne Gosling
British Federation of Care Home Proprietors

Phoebe Hall
   Observer, Department of Health

Jane Minter
   National Council for Voluntary Organisations

Alison Mitchell
   National Association of Local Government Officers

Trevor Owen CBE
   Chairman (May 1988—June 1990)

Christine Peaker
   National Council for Voluntary Organisations

Antony Pittaccio
   British Federation of Care Home Proprietors

Sheila Scott
   National Care Homes Association

Ian Sinclair
   National Institute for Social Work

Nigel Stewart
   Convention of Scottish Local Authorities

Cyril Stone
   Observer, Department of Health

Colin Vyvyan
   Observer, Welsh Office

Elizabeth Wulff-Cochrane
   Central Council for Education and Training in Social Work

CHAPTER TWO

Overview

Terry Philpot, Editor, *Community Care*

The Wagner Committee was set up after a long and seemingly unending period of neglect for residential care, with widespread anxieties about its future, poor management, and low morale among staff who were poorly paid and often untrained. Far from being the 'positive choice' which the Report's title two years later was to claim it could be, residential care was seen often as the last resort. Mostly it had failed to attract the imagination, commitment or interest of social services managers and the general swing away from residential care in favour of community-based forms of provision had made its future seem uncertain and limited. The extraordinary growth of the private sector in the first years of the 1980s gave great concern about the quality of care, standards, and fears that residents could be, or even were being, exploited for financial gain—the number of places in privately owned homes for older people and people with physical or mental disabilities nearly doubled (97 per cent) from 1979 to 1984 and by 1990 had risen by 130 per cent since 1979.[1]

The growth in the private sector had caused the care of elderly people—because it was largely they who were making use of this sector—to dominate concerns about residential care. Now, five years after the Committee's Report was published, how much has changed? Residential care has not shaken off its Cinderella status, but Wagner and subsequent reports and events have ensured that it is no longer the forgotten service. The remuneration of staff remains poor and the government has set its face against parity with field workers (unlike in Northern Ireland, where parity has been achieved).[2] The numbers of trained staff still lag lamentably behind those in fieldwork services: the Utting Report, in 1991, found that while 20 per cent of heads of children's homes were unqualified, 80 per cent of care staff lacked qualifications.[3]

However, in the intervening years concern for residential care for elderly people has given away to that for children and young people. This has come to dominate political, media and public debate. But what has been found wanting by the experience of the series of scandals that have marked residential child care is also often relevant to other areas of the residential sector.

Early on the Committee admitted its own shortcomings. It failed to include user representatives in its membership and, when the report was published, it failed to speak effectively on race.[4] The Committee also noted that it 'failed effectively to reach people with mental handicap [*sic*] and mental illness'[5] but nevertheless took extensive evidence from both carers and service providers in both these fields.

Yet, despite these drawbacks, so far as learning difficulties are concerned, the Committee has been said to have:

> . . . pointed the way to a new vision of residential care for mentally handicapped people which would only be achieved by a set of clear aims, shared philosophies and common values running throughout all provisions to be implemented and adhered to by all staff in their daily work.[6]

In the field of learning difficulties, Wagner built on earlier emphases on normalisation, notably the report of the Jay Committee in 1979.[7]

In the UK the principles of normalisation were originally taken up most strongly in this field. They are linked inextricably with the ideas of user involvement and choice, as well as matters like non-segregation and making possible patterns of living like other valued people in society. The earlier 'Home Life' code of practice had recognised this for elderly people when it said that residents of elderly people's homes 'should be involved as much as possible in making decisions concerning the way in which a home is run'.[8] But Wagner's belief that 'the needs and wishes of the user must be paramount' has been far more significant than has been recognised. For example, it predated the current preoccupation of user involvement and choice stemming from the NHS and Community Care Act 1990.

The Report said that it was written not only for politicians, policy makers and practitioners, but was addressed to a far wider audience 'for the quality of residential services affects, directly or indirectly, almost the whole population'. This itself was important, given that one commentator has called the Report 'the key publication over the past two decades' so far as 'the grassroots multi-disciplinary force with whom the practical implementation of community care policy rests' was concerned.[9]

But if the Committee had ploughed ground so constructively that had for so long remained fallow, it soon found that ground was rapidly shifting. Six months after the Committee set to work the Audit Commission published its report, 'Making a Reality of Community Care',[10] where it drew sharp attention to the method of financing places in private residential care through the social security system. This had caused a haemorrhaging of money that had pushed the bill from £6 million in 1978 to £460 million in 1988 and then to £1.3 billion in 1991.[11]

In the wake of the Report, the Secretary of State for Social Services appointed Sir Roy Griffiths to undertake his review of community care. And then midway through the Wagner Committee's two year life, disclosures were made about Nye Bevan Lodge, a south London old people's home, and these were followed in the summer by the Clough Report which looked critically at the running of homes in the London Borough of Camden.[12] These events were not exceptional as later history has proven. Scandals arising from abuse are the most dramatic symptoms of that underlying dis-ease within residential care which Wagner was setting out specifically to address.

The danger which faced the Wagner Report upon publication was less that it would be overshadowed by the scandals which were to come along with depressing regularity, but rather that its publication occurred only a few days before that of the Griffiths Report.[13] Wagner could very easily have been pushed to the back of the queue as the political spotlight shone upon Sir Roy's recommendations for a fundamental shift for local authorities from being providers to purchasers of services from the independent (private and voluntary) sector. This would be (it was said) the way of improving services, creating real choice for users, and tailoring services to meet their specific needs. In November 1989 the Department of Health published its response to Griffiths in a White Paper 'Caring for People',[14] which within a year was translated into the National Health Service and Community Care Act.

But while much attention did focus on Griffiths, two major important consequences relevant to Wagner's concerns arose from the legislation which Griffiths had engendered. The first was that from 1 April 1993 social security monies which would have been available to support people in private and voluntary residential care were ring fenced and transferred to social services departments, who then had the responsibility of making an assessment to see whether residential care or care in the community was most appropriate. (The position of those residents already in residential care with the support of state funds was protected). Second, with the new purchaser/provider split, local authorities began to hive off much of their residential provision, especially that for elderly people, as self-governing trusts, or into the hands of private owners or as a result of management buy-outs.

Wagner did not bring about a public discussion or attract political attention to rival anything achieved by Griffiths, 'Caring for People', and the passing of the legislation through Parliament. While some of its recommendations (for example number 28 that made local authority, voluntary and private residential establishments subject to the same system of legislation and inspection, and number 34 on the registration of small homes) were taken onto the statute book, the revolution which it had foreseen was not enshrined in legislation, as was the Griffiths Report. Thus, much of what it wanted might have suffered the slow death by neglect which is so often the notorious lot of inquiry reports but for three things. First, the Wagner Development Group was set up, under the aegis of the National Institute for Social Work, to take forward the Report's ideas and recommendations. As Sir Kenneth Stowe commented:

> Because it is so remarkable, unprecedented and uplifting in this context, I cite as a right attitude, Lady Wagner's Committee in setting up its own post-report development group of all interested parties to bring about, without authority and without government money, the betterment in residential care that is so much desired.[15]

The Development Group broke into specialist Sub-Groups to look at issues like quality assurance; black perspectives; security of tenure and tenants' rights (where it drew up a code of practice); complaints procedures; residential child care (to produce a charter for children); and staffing arrangements. One of its first tasks was to draw up a checklist of ten points of good practice, from the Report, that could immediately be acted upon in all sectors across the whole span of residential care and which would not have major resource implications. These points included a brochure or prospectus setting out an establishment's aims and objectives; written contracts on the rights of residents; complaints procedures; a strategy to abolish stigmatising practices like the issuing of order forms to residents to buy items like clothes and food; and providing staff with proper induction, supervision and appropriate training opportunities.

The list also included procedures to recognise and deal with the fact that residents' rights are limited for their own and other people's safety, and to ensure at least six monthly reviews of services for residents whose abilities to make decisions are limited. The checklist also stressed the desirability of policies on equal opportunities for staff, regular meetings for staff, an annual review of the home's aims and objectives and practices, and the recruitment of staff able to listen to residents, to understand what they say and to see them as individuals in a social context rather than as members of disadvantaged groups.

The Group's work was pushed forward by the issuing of a regular newsletter, and by its holding four major national conferences in association with 'Community Care'. The first of these, 'Wagner: The Residential Opportunity', effectively launched the Report in April 1988 and was attended by 450 people, a sign that residential care was truly on the social services agenda. From this conference came a book.[16] The other conferences followed in October 1989, November 1991, and April 1993.

The second engine that powered a continuing interest in the Report was the establishment by the government of the Caring in Homes Initiative, launched in February 1989 as a £2.2 million, three-year programme to assist individual staff, owners, residents, managers and others at a practical level to improve the quality of life in their homes. It gave especial emphasis to four important aspects of residential care, with materials being produced by four different agencies:

—providing information to residents, potential residents and carers (Policy Studies Institute);

—involving residents in evaluating and improving the quality of life in their home (Centre for Environmental and Social Studies at the University of North London);

—staff development training (National Institute for Social Work);

—Window in Homes: linking homes and the wider community (Social Care Association Education)

(The Initiative is discussed fully by Penny Youll in Chapter Eight.)

The third factor in keeping Wagner alive and well was some of the very issues which had brought the Committee into being in the first place: the seemingly endemically poor state of residential services, resulting in a series of scandals (most often in the child care sector) which spawned inquiries that continued to find poor management, abuse, poor communications, and low levels of training. (In Staffordshire, however, the practice of pindown was carried out by staff with impeccable social work qualifications. In Leicestershire, the trial of Frank Beck revealed years of physical and sexual abuse by an equally well-qualified practitioner.)

Both Staffordshire and Leicestershire showed serious failures in communications within the departments, as well as poor management. The Utting Report,[18] commissioned in the wake of pindown, was specifically charged to consider management and monitoring. Its chief recommendation was that the head of every children's home should be qualified by 1996 (Wagner had said 1993). The Report also recommended that the arm's length inspection units of social services departments must regularly inspect all an authority's children's homes. Furthermore, the Central Council for Education and Training in Social Work, the local authority associations and the Department of Health should devise a training strategy for all staff—though the Report's author, Sir William Utting, admitted he was not able to assess training needs—within five years.

His Report's other recommendations included the inspection of all voluntary homes; the approval of all types of secure accommodation by the Secretary of State; guidance by local authorities on the roles of members in the running of homes; and the management of all a home's resources by heads of homes. The Secretary of State promised to implement all the recommendations. She also said that she could make no financial commitment.

Utting offered some way forward. But he did not find the crux of the crisis to be poor pay and conditions for workers, but bad management above them. Here he underpinned the concerns of the earlier Levy/Kahan Report on pindown in Staffordshire, though in not emphasising pay and conditions as a factor, he was in disagreement with that Report.[19] Utting was helpful, however, in repeating Wagner's emphasis that residential care was here to stay, an acceptable and accepted part of the total spectrum of care, though his Report failed to clearly spell out residents' rights and how to protect them, as Wagner had done.

When in June 1992 the Howe inquiry into pay and conditions, training and qualifications reported,[20] it was sandwiched between the Utting Report and the then expected Warner Report,[21] which had been set up in the wake of the Beck case in Leicestershire. But Howe provided an unofficial framework for negotiations and had won a package on pay and conditions for residential workers. It did not neglect training, repeating some of Wagner's ideas, while adding new ideas of its own. It called for an induction programme of basic training for all new staff (thus pursuing one of the ideas which had emerged from the CHI). It repeated previous calls that local authorities should draw up training plans, adding that National Vocational Qualifications units should be used to develop in-house training courses.

Like Utting, it saw proper management training as a key to tackling both managerial problems generally, and more specifically poor staff morale. Howe listed 30 recommendations. These inevitably had resource implications, but like Utting, Howe played these down: its justification for spending was that it was cost effective. Howe was generally greeted with support coupled by a belief that it—like other reports—needed cash on the table if it was to be successful.

Six months later the Warner Report, deriving from the Beck scandal in Leicestershire, was published. Now, it was less a case of the local authorities seeking to nudge the Department of Health into action, more the Department giving local authorities six months to implement several of the Report's 83 recommendations. The Department issued a circular to accompany the Report's publication to this effect. Warner was concerned with recruitment and staff selection, but specifically addressed situations whereby sexual abusers were able to find themselves jobs working with vulnerable young people. Among other things, Warner wanted a review of complaints procedures (Wagner had recommended them, and they had been established, for children, under the Children Act 1989); fortnightly staff supervision; personal development contracts; new recruitment techniques; independent counselling and support for staff; needs-led plans; a review of the independent visiting service for homes; and external advertising for staff. Most controversially, Warner wanted a review of equal opportunities policies, believing that a too rigid adherence to them had made it difficult to probe suitability to work in residential child care.

The Report did not place all the responsibility on local authorities: from government it wanted a national directory of children's homes; new codes of good practice and employment practice; pump-priming initiatives on recruitment techniques; and training line managers for appraisal and supervision, backed by a national training strategy. Warner found staff untrained, poorly managed and supervised. Extra training demanded additional funding.

The Report also recommended a separate residential child care qualification. But the idea of a separate qualification (albeit Warner had placed an emphasis on work-related training) found few supporters. With the old Certificate of Qualification in Social Work not long merged with the Certificate in Social Service to create the new single qualification, the Diploma in Social Work, Warner's suggestion seemed like a resuscitation of the CSS or a step back even further to the days before CQSW and the CSS with a variety of qualifications in child care and residential work. However, considerably in favour of a separate qualification was the fact that DipSW's curriculum was chock full already of, arguably, too many subjects, each dealt with in no great depth, so that the introduction of any child care option would only aggravate that condition. The junior Health Minister, Tim Yeo, warned that 'a variety of weapons' would be available to the government if authorities did not meet the 8 April deadline to implement the recommendations, but he refused to be drawn on extra funding.[22]

Soon after the Wagner Development Group met for the last time, two more reports on the Beck case—the government inquiry by Andrew Kirkwood QC and one by the police—appeared.[23] Kirkwood, confirming a sad history from Wagner to Warner, found a 'management vacuum' in Leicestershire. The need for the residential child care development group, which Warner had urged upon government, seemed all the more urgent in the light of Kirkwood's findings.

It would be wrong to see Kirkwood, which was investigating events which had taken place over 13 years, as a sad epitaph to Wagner and subsequent events and reports. Much had changed even since Beck had been sentenced: the review of the first year of the Children Act[24] had shown that fewer children were being taken into compulsory care (though not all of those who were would have gone into residential care). But first appraisal of the Act had also shown confusion still on the part of local authorities about what they should do in the face of allegations of abuse in a residential home.

Wagner was the most comprehensive review of residential care for 20 years. Unlike earlier reports, like that of the Curtis Committee,[25] it had also been concerned with the whole range of client groups. There were those who have questioned its fundamental premise that residential care can be a part of the community[26] or can be a positive choice, as opposed to admission to residential care being something that takes place in crisis.[27] But Wagner had established, both in its Report and through the work of the Development Group, that residential care was not only central to the agenda of welfare provision—be it for elderly people or young people—but that it can have a future.

Many issues about training, not least the vast training needs which remain unmet, remain unresolved. Positively, the shift of the Central Council for Education and Training in Social Work, in response to the urgings of the expert group set up after Utting, that DIPSW courses should treat residential care 'as central to mainstream social work',[28] was another confirmation of Wagner's wisdom.

Wagner proved its worth by focusing attention on residential care across the range of client need, in its recommendations, and in the work of the Development Group. It also stood as a reference point and measure very often for what came after it. This is where the value of its comprehensiveness showed: from inquiries into abuse, management, or pay and conditions, it could be a marker.

Those who take a negative view might point less to how much has changed, but to how much remains regrettably the same, of which each new scandal or report seems too tangible a confirmation. Residential care continues to journey in a long, dark tunnel. The glimpses of light at the end are very rare. Wagner can be credited with having created enough ways through which that light may find a way.

Notes

1. Alan Walker, 'Community care policy: From consensus to conflict', in Joanna Barnet, Charmaine Pereria, David Pilgrim and Fiona Williams (editors), *Community Care: A Reader*, Open University/Macmillan, 1992.
2. Will Hatchett, 'The Irish route to parity', *Community Care*, 15 September, 1991.
3. Sir William Utting, *Children in the Public Care*, HMSO, 1991.
4. For three views of Wagner's consideration of race see Viola Nzira, Julia Phillipson and Mary Sugden; Viola Nzira; and Ben Brown in Terry Philpot (editor), *The Residential Opportunity? The Wagner Report and After*, Community Care/Reed Business Publishing, 1989.

5. Independent Review into Residential Care (Wagner Committee), *Residential Care: A Positive Choice*, HMSO, 1988.

6. Janice C. Sinson, *Group Homes and Community Integration of Developmentally Disabled People. Micro-Institutionalisation?*, Jessica Kingsley Publishers, 1993.

7. Jay Committee, *Report into the Committee of Inquiry into Mental Handicap Nursing and Care*, HMSO, 1979. See also, David Towell (editor), *An Ordinary Life: Comprehensive, Locally Based Residential Services for Mentally Handicapped People*, King's Fund Centre, 1980 and the subsequent *Ordinary Life* series.

8. Avebury Committee, *Home Life: A Code of Practice for Residential Care*, Centre for Policy on Ageing, 1984.

9. Sinson, *op. cit.*

10. HMSO, 1986.

11. Walker, *op. cit.*

12. London Borough of Camden, *Independent Review of Residential Care for Elderly People in the London Borough of Camden*, 1987.

13. Sir Roy Griffiths, *Community Care: Agenda for Action*, HMSO, 1988.

14. DoH, *Caring for People: Community Care in the Decade and Beyond*, HMSO, 1989.

15. Sir Kenneth Stowe, *On Caring for the National Health*, Nuffield Provincial Hospitals Trust, 1989.

16. Philpot (editor), *op. cit.*

17. Ruth Elkan and Des Kelly, *A Window in Homes: Links Between Residential Care Homes and the Community. A Literature Review*, Social Care Association, 1991.

18. Utting, *op. cit.*

19. Alan Levy and Barbara Kahan, *The Pindown Experience and the Protection of Children. Report of the Staffordshire Child Care Inquiry 1990*, Staffordshire County Council, 1991.

20. Howe Committee, *The Quality of Care: Report of the Residential Staff Inquiry*, Local Government Management Board, 1992.

21. Norman Warner, *Choosing with Care*, HMSO, 1992.

22. Bob Cervi, 'Government calls for early implementation of Warner', *Community Care*, 10 December, 1992.

23. Andrew Kirkwood, *The Leicestershire Inquiry 1992*, Leicestershire County Council, 1993; and summary of the police report, Police Complaints Commission, 1993.

24. DoH and the Welsh Office, *The Childen Act Report, 1992*, HMSO, 1993.

25. Curtis Committee, *Report of the Care of Child Committee*, HMSO, 1946.
26. See Chris Hanvey, 'A sign of the times', *Community Care*, 22 August 1991.
27. See Walker, *op. cit.* who also quotes Bradshaw as concluding that the promise of choice is illusory. (Jonathan Bradshaw, *Financing Private Care for the Elderly*, Department of Social Policy and Social Work, University of York, 1988).
28. Central Council for Education and Training in Social Work, *Residential Child Care in the Diploma in Social Work*, 1992.

The author would like to thank the following for their comments and suggestions: Dick Clough, General Secretary, Social Care Association; Chris Hanvey, Director, Thomas Coram Foundation; John Pierson, freelance trainer and teacher; and Linda Ward, Senior Research Fellow, Norah Fry Research Centre, University of Bristol.

Rights, Responsibilities, Relationships and Regulations

David C. Lane, Wakefield Community and Social Services
Department

Introduction

There is confusion at present both in thinking and in practice concerning the rights of people in residential care. This chapter is intended to clarify some of the confusions and give pointers for action.

By way of example, the Wagner Report rightly emphasises the need for residential care to be a positive choice, and yet, without legal backing, staff lock the doors of homes for the elderly to contain those who wish to get out. Again, there is a drive to maintain young people in their local communities, currently offset by a drive to lock up those involved in taking and driving cars. Or again, there are the many subtle pressures placed upon residents to conform, to please staff, and to make life easier for staff, which may be in opposition to the ways in which the residents wish to live, or which may detract from the opportunities they need to realise their potential.

What rights do residents have in practice? What rights should they have? And what should be done about it?

Four Levels of Questioning

These questions need to be answered simultaneously at several levels if the problems are to be resolved:

—at the **practical** level, the day-to-day life of residential homes needs to reflect policy, law and theory on rights;

—at the **policy** level, agencies need guidelines which make sense in practice, which are consistent with the law, and which reflect sound fundamental thinking on rights;

—at the **legal** level, laws need to support good practice and reflect sound fundamental thinking; and

—at the **theoretical** level, thinking needs to reflect the right values and attitudes, and needs to be able to stand up to questioning in terms of ethics and moral philosophy.

If either thinking or practice at any of the four levels is inconsistent, then residents are liable to suffer the consequences. Indeed, at present, not only do residents pay the penalty for shortcomings in our present state of thinking and practice, but so do staff.

Modes of Relating

The use of the term 'rights' implies a certain way of looking at relationships. Just as in the days before Hammurabi and Moses with their codified laws there were no doubt unwritten laws by which people lived as an accepted code of behaviour, similarly people have enjoyed rights before they were identified, debated and written down. Rights have been expressed by being exercised, and assumptions were made that they existed, for example in legislation, before attempts were made to identify them and define them.

In defining rights, relationships between people are circumscribed. If everyone is granted the right to free speech, for example, everyone is also denied the right to prevent others speaking freely. As society has become more sophisticated, we have come to accept more and more limitations on our behaviour through laws, regulations, written codes of behaviour and unwritten social conduct, in order to be able to enjoy freedoms that make the limitations worthwhile.

The definition of rights is therefore part of a complex process of social negotiation, and it expresses an intention to preserve the freedoms people feel are of greatest importance, worth designating, and worth trading limitations for.

Problems of Definition

The process of definition is, of course, a human activity. Determining what constitutes a right is up to those involved. Definitions may be tight or loose, as people wish. The focus of a right may be specific, or broad and general. For example, one may seek the right to vote, or the right to participate in democratic politics. The consequences of the way rights are defined are clearly considerable.

Rights are therefore human constructs. They do not have a platonic ideal existence. Some people have described rights as 'inalienable'; even at the theoretical level, this is nonsense, while at the practical level, clearly rights can be taken away from people.

This does not mean that rights are at all unimportant. Respect for the rights of individuals or groups is of vital importance. Where they are infringed or treated as unimportant, there is a serious danger of abuse, for example in the treatment of Jews as 'unter-menchen' in Hitler's Germany. We live in an age when we are finding it necessary to clarify and define many aspects of our social behaviour, and it is particularly important that people who are powerless or vulnerable should have their freedoms preserved.

While there are certain sections of society which are more vulnerable than others, such as the very frail, the confused and the seriously disabled—indeed, nearly all people in residential care—it will be evident that all of us could find ourselves vulnerable at some stage of our lives, and it is therefore a matter of self-interest as well as altruism that the way rights are defined protects vulnerable people.

Rights and Power

The definition of rights concerns the distribution of power, and consciously gives control to people who are powerless and vulnerable, taking it from those who would otherwise be in control because of their roles, status or control of resources.

There have been many occasions in history when a subjugated section of the people have demanded rights and the matter has been resolved by politics or force. By and large, people in residential care homes are unable to be their own advocates, and they have neither the strength nor the resources to challenge the power of those in charge. Indeed, analysis of scandals has regularly shown that residents conform through fear even when their rights have been seriously eroded.

It is therefore evident that if a fundamental value of our society is that the individuality of people is to be respected and that they are to be treated as being of worth (ie with dignity), then regardless of the factors that make them vulnerable, extra effort will be needed from those who are not vulnerable, particularly if they are in positions of power, to help to protect people who are vulnerable, among other things by defining their rights, and ensuring that they are implemented.

Indeed, there are strong arguments for residents, especially when they are vulnerable or unable to argue on their own behalf, having advocates to speak on their behalf. This role was recognised in the Wagner Report and is reflected in child care legislation. It is particularly important where there is fear of subsequent recriminations against residents, which can leave both them and their relatives under pressure to keep quiet about unacceptable standards.

Choice and Control

In choosing 'A Positive Choice' as the title of its Report, the Wagner Committee gave a number of messages. One of them was that entering and living in residential care should entail choice, which implies that someone has the power to choose.

The umbrella title included residents, potential residents and their families among the choosers, choosing not only whether to make use of residential care, or which home to select, but also how to live day-by-day in the home. This implied that residents and those concerned for them should have real control, and that there should be a shift in power from the authorities and the staff to those whom the services are meant to serve.

This shift is consistent with the fundamental value mentioned above: that individuals are each of worth and even when vulnerable must be treated with dignity. Interestingly, the same value is implicit in the approach to assessment and care management taken in 'Care in the Community' planning, in which people are assisted to define their own needs and ways in which they may be met, giving them as much choice as possible within the resources available.

Negotiation

It should be noted that all these processes entail negotiation. Because the rights of the people involved are defined by people, there are no absolutes, and social interaction is required to determine what is best in the circumstances.

Some rights may be agreed by all involved as being fixed of course, and these may be enshrined in law or regulations. Others may be less firm, as evidenced in guidelines, or may be enunciated as principles to be balanced against other conflicting principles in decision-making.

It is not the purpose of this chapter to draw up model rights for residents. This could no doubt be done, whether for the guidance of individual responsible agencies or for national acceptance; but it must be noted that even if a core set of rights were established, there would always be others applying to individual homes, or which were adopted in some circumstances and then abandoned when circumstances changed. To be relevant and real, rights need to be continually renegotiated, in order to reflect current concerns and relationships and to ensure that the worth and dignity of the individuals involved is reinforced.

It is of great importance to recognise and accept the need for continual renegotiation for two reasons. First, there is the danger that rights come to be seen as something rigid, fixed and unchangeable. Life, and relationships with other people, are changeable and dynamic. The mechanisms we use to manage our relationships, and the language and concepts we use, therefore need to be similarly malleable, live and dynamic. If not, the language, concepts and mechanisms may themselves take control and stultify the relationships and lives of those involved.

Secondly, there is the danger that people who see the importance of rights and the critical need to protect the vulnerable by emphasising rights set up a kind of crusade to battle on behalf of the underdog, and in the process blind themselves to the fact that people are not just individuals living in isolation, but are social individuals living in a network of bonds and relationships, which may be internalised and contribute to the shaping of the individual. Removed from the network and placed in another, the individual responds differently.

The significance of this line of argument is that the rights crusader, basing his/her thinking on the value of people as individuals, would see any infringement of individual rights as something wrong, to be combated. But if one sees rights as only one aspect of our social relationships, acknowledging that the giving of rights means also the giving up of rights, then the issue is seen in a more complex context, including personal responsibilities for example, among other aspects of relating.

Following this line of argument, there are three types of grounds which may justify the diminution of an individual's rights.

Choosing to Give Up Rights

First, it is acceptable for individuals to give up their rights voluntarily. The classic example is of the monk taking a vow of poverty, chastity and obedience and entering a life of silent contemplation, giving up the rights of life in the wider society for personal spiritual purposes.

At a much more modest level, any person choosing to enter a residential care home will know that their life will be in some way constrained by the nature of group living, the needs of other residents, and the needs of the staff. There may cease to be a choice of mealtimes or menus, perhaps, or one may have to compromise about how one keeps possessions even in one's bedroom, for the sake of the cleaners and hygiene standards.

Any limitations of the sort described above should be known to potential residents and their families so that a choice can be made, whether it is better to accept the loss of certain freedoms for the gains from living in the home. The Caring in Homes Initiative 'Information for Users' programme lays out this issue.

Clearly, people often take up places in residential care homes in order to make life easier for carers, and there can be many hidden pressures underlying such decisions. In good practice, these pressures should be made explicit, acknowledged and considered in forming balanced judgements which take account of all the factors involved. Hopefully the assessment processes involved in Care in the Community will encourage good practice, which will lay sounder foundations for residents' experience of care, and their relationships with their relatives and carers.

Changes made once people are resident present a different problem in terms of choice, and should be subject to negotiation with those involved so that they can decide on the response they wish to make to proposed changes.

Incapacity

Secondly, there are individuals who are incapable of making the full range of choices normally handled by people in the community. Individuals in this group may be severely mentally disabled or severely confused, or again, they may be very young. These people lose their rights in practice, and their families and staff simply take decisions about them. Such practice is justifiable insofar as the people in question are demonstrably unable to exercise judgement.

The presumption has always to be made that people are capable of choice and control over their own lives unless it is clear that they cannot take on this responsibility, however, for three reasons. First, the basic principle should be that individuals control their own lives and it should be the rare exception that rights should be diminished on the grounds of incapacity. Secondly, where people may become more independent, the pressure should be exerted to give them progressively more control over their own lives and a presumption should always be made in favour of taking calculated risks in order to give wider scope to the person instead of playing safe and being unduly protective. Thirdly, because of the power of their positions, there is always the dangerous tendency for family members and staff to take control, even for the best of reasons, and this therefore has to be continually checked and tested.

The problem is much more acute in relation to people who are capable of a certain level of decision-making but who nonetheless put themselves at risk at times, or who have periods of lucidity and periods of emotional imbalance. This group includes some people recovering from mental illnesses, for example, or disturbed adolescents. The principles outlined above remain the same, but are much more difficult to apply, and it is here that many of today's dilemmas are seen most acutely.

It is not possible legally to restrain adolescents in care from absconding, offending or indulging in sexual behaviour unless there is justification for placing them in secure accommodation. Yet many people clearly feel that residential staff are failing if they do not contain behaviour generally deemed anti-social or unacceptable.

Similarly, adults may wish to exercise their rights to live independently in squalor or to behave oddly. Society often expects social services intervention when there are no legal grounds, and influence is limited to persuasion based on the strength of relationships between staff and residents.

In most of these cases, neither families nor staff have any right in law to curtail the freedoms of residents, regardless of their ability to take decisions and have control over their own lives. Yet there is a clear expectation on the part of the public that placement in residential care will provide a degree of protection and containment, and that staff will be failing if it is not provided.

In the event, there are times, particularly in residential child care, when the behaviour is not contained, and there is local reaction to the resulting anti-social behaviour and offending. There are also times when staff go beyond their legal rights: for example in the containment of confused elderly wanderers. The nub of the problem is that staff and residents are both in a legal limbo, where rights and responsibilities are left unclear.

Deprivation of Rights

The third justification for diminishing residents' rights is that, in response to their own behaviour, they need to be deprived of them. This is essentially a problem of delinquency and criminality, although it also applies to some behaviour problems or mental health issues.

If a person is a danger to others, to him/herself, or to property, there may well be grounds for containment and the associated loss of rights. Examples include murderers, arsonists, people involved in taking and driving away cars, people who damage themselves or leave themselves vulnerable through habitual absconding. On the child care front, these people are the population of secure units. As adults, many are in prisons and mental hospitals, but some are also in residential care, for example in probation hostels.

Although the two groups overlap at certain points, for example when disturbed children are in residential care, the justification for the third group being deprived of their rights is substantially different from the second group. The second should enjoy whatever rights they can cope with; the third is specifically told by society, often formally through the courts, that their behaviour is unacceptable and that they therefore have to forego their rights.

Clearly there is an important overlap, in that demonstration of the ability to exercise proper control over their own lives may satisfy society to allow residents in the third category to be freed of the constraints placed upon them. Similarly, residents' anti-social behaviour could be read as grounds for deeming them incapable of proper decision-making and choice.

The distinction however has to be acknowledged: curtailment of the rights of the second group is essentially in their own interest and has no other justification, whereas the third group's diminution of rights is authorised by society and may be in the interests of others. In the practice of residential care it is important for all concerned to be honest and clear about this distinction.

The Rights of Others

The main emphasis of discussions about rights quite properly focuses mainly upon residents, because it is their rights which usually suffer erosion. However, other people involved also have rights, including residents' families, staff, staff families, and the neighbours of a home. Some of these relate to the specific roles played by these people, but others relate to the common humanity we all share, and the rights we should all have.

Just as residents should not have to suffer loss of rights simply because of their vulnerability, so staff should not lose their rights simply because their chosen role is to be of service to the residents. For example, where residents are capable of being responsible for their own behaviour, there is no reason for staff to suffer assault at the hands of residents without the right of redress, just as residents should be equally protected.

As discussed earlier, the actual definition and exercise of rights in any one home will need to be a matter of negotiation. The resident's right to stay up late may well entail the staff loss of right to get to bed or go home. Exercising the right to play loud music in one's room may impact on the neighbourhood. There are daily examples of conflicts of this sort, none of which have absolute answers, and they require negotiation between the interested parties, with a view to achieving a mutually acceptable compromise which infringes the rights of those involved as little as possible.

Responsibilities

At the most naive level of thinking, people argue for rights to be observed, without any consideration of responsibilities. At another level, responsibilities are seen as the other side of the coin of rights. This thinking has its attractions, in that people earn their rights by carrying out their responsibilities (no representation without taxation!), and it is the basis of token economy treatment systems.

However, rights and responsibilities, although both aspects of the way we relate to each other, are not mirrored opposites, and there is a danger of being simplistic in seeing them in this light.

In the field of residential care there are broadly three types of responsibility. The first and most obvious is that of the staff, who are paid to carry accountability for the duties they perform as laid out in their job descriptions. Their role is fundamentally formal. They can be expected to carry out what is required of them, and if they fail to do so, they can be disciplined or dismissed. They are expected to continue to be of service, even if they are unmotivated, and they have compensating rights to pay and other benefits which are not enjoyed by other people who may play similar roles, such as volunteers.

The second type of responsibility is that of the family. Whether because of close and early contact or for genetic reasons, family ties are usually seen as overriding other types of relationships, with strong bonds of mutual responsibility: blood is thicker than water.

Interestingly, relationships of this closeness often build up in residential care, as well as in fostering or adoption, where it might be expected. Staff may come to be seen as family by residents, and vice versa. For children in care, these ties can continue throughout adult life.

Responsibilities of this type cannot be required of anyone, and if accepted, have to be taken on voluntarily. Residents cannot therefore claim a right to such a level of relationship. If staff and residents come to feel a level of mutual commitment of this type, it is well beyond the minimalist demands of rights.

Indeed it is interesting that many measures adopted by agencies are actually designed to combat the problems that may arise when relationships between staff and residents are seen to be too close and not in the residents' interests. These include the forbidding of sexual relationships between staff and residents, regulations to prevent residents leaving money to staff, and warnings against the danger of staff becoming over-involved emotionally.

Clearly residents need to be protected from exploitation by the people appointed to protect, support and care for them, but the measures taken to avoid such exploitation may also deprive residents at times of really close and rewarding relationships.

The third type of responsibility is that of all people for each other; society is not simply made of individuals, but we are all bound together in a complex web of relationships, including an element of mutual responsibility. It is seen in the social conduct we expect of each other, in mutual help at times of accident or crisis, and in the acceptance of mechanisms, such as the legal system, for dealing with aberrations from the norm.

In residential care, residents often care for staff, or for each other, and the resident group as a whole can be a powerful force for influencing its members to behave in particular ways, for good or ill.

In the residential setting therefore, everyone has some rights and some responsibilities. Everyone's freedoms are limited to some extent, and insofar as people have chosen to be resident or have acknowledged that they are members of the residential community, they adopt those limitations as a matter of choice. However, these need to stand as key principles—that rights are diminished as little as possible, and that there is no general loss of rights, only the removal of specified rights for specified challengeable reasons.

Any definition of the rights of residents and othe responsibilities of staff has therefore to be set in a wider and more complex context. To emphasise rights on their own reduces people to being considered only as individuals, when in fact much of the significance of their lives lies in their familial and social interactions. Discussion about rights must therefore take account of people's social behaviour. To ignore the context will result in a naive definition of rights and responsiblities which will not work in practice and will detract from the lives of both residents and staff.

Where Next?

The issue of residents' rights has to be debated more widely. It needs to be analysed and discussed in every qualifying training course, in every agency and in every home. The common features of every major scandal in residential care are the abuse of power by staff and the vulnerability of the residents.

Discussion about residents' rights will focus the work on the prime purpose of residential care, to serve the residents' needs. This is necessary in every home. Scandals are only a symptom of the worst aspects of rights abuse. A much greater problem is the insidious erosion of rights on a daily basis, perhaps unwittingly on the part of staff, who may have the best of intentions.

Where residents have choices made for them which they can make for themselves, where the smooth running of a home is essentially staff-centred, where residents are deprived of opportunities to develop by the way the home is being run, their rights are being denied. This is happening in homes that are happy and well run. Their practice may well be good, but it is not good enough. A good test is whether residents actually exercise the freedoms stated about the running of the home.

What is more, the questioning on these issues should be never-ending. Observing residents' rights is not something one can tick off on the checklist as being done and finished with. It is part of the ongoing dynamics of life in homes, because there is the perpetual tension between the power of the staff, the vulnerability of the residents, and the ways in which their rights are justifiably diminished. This is not simply a matter of staff awareness, though. The staff work in a faulty legal and managerial context, which leaves them unsupported for the duties they have to take on.

The three ways in which rights may be diminished give a pointer for the action required. First, in terms of the voluntary loss of rights which arises from being a member of a residential community, the situation should be spelt out in every single home so that everyone involved—residents, potential residents, their families, staff, other members of the agency and even the public—know what is entailed. When contracting to enter residential care, along with taking on the tenancy, a resident needs to know what is entailed in admission, both the benefits and the limitations, so that an open and conscious choice can be made, with which s/he can identify and carry the responsibility for fulfilling his/her role. This action can be taken within existing practice, and is consistent with all recent legislation.

The second type of diminution of rights, on grounds of the incapacity of residents, presents the main problem, since practice and expectations both deviate from the letter of the law significantly. Again, this will best be dealt with by making the issues explicit. If residents lack the capacity to enjoy certain rights, for example by being unable to make decisions or choices, then this needs to be spelt out as part of their care plan, and acknowledged in the care contract.

If, for example, a person is too confused to be allowed out on busy roads alone, the contract may state that accompanied walks would be arranged, but that the resident would otherwise be kept in the home. To avoid the charge that this process would make serious inroads into residents' rights, it would have to be open ultimately to appeal to the courts, either by residents themselves or by other people on their behalf, although it is hoped that such appeals would be exceptional.

In some circumstances staff might wish to argue that they could not offer care without limitations to a resident's rights, and this argument too could be tested in the courts, if necessary.

The advantages of such a system are that:

—it would make all diminutions of rights explicit relating to individuals, who should otherwise enjoy their full rights as citizens within the residential community;

—it would give staff the explicit authority to act where residents were known to be incapable of exercising proper judgement, instead of their current uncertainty;

—it would be readily grafted on to other systems of care planning, as described in the Children Act 1989, and the National Health Service and Community Care Act 1990;

—it would be accountable to the courts and therefore challenge-able, while not making excessive additional demands, since most of this work would be undertaken as part of the normal social services assessment and care planning processes.

The third type of diminution of rights relates to the deprivation of rights on the grounds of anti-social, delinquent or criminal behaviour. This is mainly conducted through the courts, and there are systems available therefore for dealing with matters of this sort.

However, it could be argued that in one important respect, the powers required are at present inadequate. Particularly in the field of child care, there are types of behaviour such as absconding, pilfering and taking and driving cars, which warrant action in order to prevent them, but where placement in secure accommodation is seen as inappropriate, being excessively punitive or liable to lead to inappropriate contacts or self-images. Other measures, such as curfews, tracking or restrictions on young people's liberty during remand, are available, but have not been used much. The use of semi-secure provision has not found favour because of the danger that young people's rights would be at risk of being subject to the whims of staff.

However, it is clear that for a comparatively small group of young people, the present measures are seen as inadequate at present, and if punitive measures are to be avoided, there is need for a wider and more informed debate on measures that are effective, so that the wider community feels protected and so that young people do not build up records of delinquency and antisocial behaviour as a result of the system's failures.

If measures were permissible which contained young people's behaviour short of secure placement, histories of offending and considerable anguish on the part of the young people's victims might be avoided. Such measures could be handled through care planning systems similar to the proposals for dealing with residents incapable of dealing with their own decisions outlined above, but it is possible that these measures should be part of the courts' range of decisions, as being part of the justice system.

It will be seen that these proposals entail legislation, but without it, the situation will remain confused. Residents will remain without explicit protection, and staff will remain open to criticism for failing in their duties or for overstepping the mark.

CHAPTER FOUR

Aspects of Quality in Residential Care

Sub-Group Report

Introduction

The Sub-Group on a Quality Assurance matters was given the remit to take forward the thinking behind the SCA/ADSS document 'Standard Setting in the Personal Social Services'; other remits were added throughout the life of the Sub-Group, which by 1992 had changed its title to the more accurate description of 'Aspects of Quality in Residential Care'.

The Sub-Group commenced its work in two specific ways. The first task was to use the 'Standard Setting' paper to examine to what extent a checklist model of inspection could be developed; the second task was to take each of the recommendations in the Wagner Report which referred to quality of life opportunities in residential care and to consider what action, if any, was required to promote the intention of the recommendation.

In reporting on the work of the Quality Assurance Sub-Group, the question which arises must be 'To what extent was the Wagner Report a causative factor in the development of aspects of quality in much subsequent work?' It is unlikely that many will challenge that the work of the Sub-Group encouraged many and prompted the pursuance of new work which might not have happened without the underpinning resolve of the Wagner Development Group to 'see something done'.

The work done by the Sub-Group around the issue of using a checklist approach to inspection in a residential setting is reported in Section 2 of this report. Section 1 examines each of the Wagner recommendations which reflected upon quality issues. The task has been frustrating at times (as the results of other work were awaited), sometimes challenging (as the Sub-Group investigated new initiatives), but always worthwhile. Recording our conclusions maintains this rich mixture.

Section One

'Ensuring the Quality of Residential Services' Monitored

Response to the Wagner Recommendations on Quality

'A Positive Choice' contains a chapter entitled 'Ensuring the Quality of Residential Services'. Each of these recommendations was addressed.

1. LOCAL AUTHORITIES SHOULD TAKE THE LEAD IN THE STRATEGIC PLANNING OF RESIDENTIAL SERVICES

This concept is now integrated into the National Health Service and Community Care Act 1990, in which each local authority is required to 'prepare and publish a plan for the provision of community care services in their area', keep the plan under review, and publish modifications as necessary. In the preparation of such a plan, a local authority must consult with appropriate health authorities, housing authorities, and voluntary and private sector organisations.

This development was warmly welcomed by the Wagner Development Group as it confirms the philosophy underpinning both Wagner and Griffiths, and places lead responsibility in strategic planning of services with the local authority. At a time when local authorities believed themselves to be under siege by central government through inadequate funding, rate capping, the consequences of the community charge, and the threat of removal of power through the use of specific grants, social services departments were pleasantly pleased to be given this lead responsibility. The Department of Health and its counterparts in the other countries of the United Kingdom have issued extensive direction and guidance on what must be done; it should be recorded that the spirit of such writings has been directed at cost effective but quality assured services.

The inclusion of residential care in the wider range of community care services continues, and confirms the Wagner philosophy of choice. It is to be hoped that the counter-balances of individual care packages using specific budget holders and the possibility of the local authority purchasing a 'block of beds' will be sustained to the benefit and needs of the individual. Just as the Act gives the local authority many opportunities to advance the quality issues identified in Wagner, it is possible for financial reasons to fail to maximise the full potential of the Act.

Health authorities carry responsibility for the strategic planning of health care services. Health and local authorities are urged to co-operate in the formulation of joint planning agreements and, where feasible, joint community care plans. Again, government circulars continue to emphasise the potential for positive practice.

In April 1993, the responsibility for funding residential care, including nursing care, passed to the local authorities. This is further confirmation of the lead responsibility of local authorities.

The work of the Black Perspectives Sub-Group is reported upon elsewhere, but in the context of quality in residential care, it is appropriate to draw attention to the recommendations and implications of the work of that Sub-Group. Local authorities have taken the lead in pursuing the qualities of equal opportunity employers, and this is a further opportunity to listen to a minority group view.

The Quality Assurance Sub-Group has been involved individually—and often directly as a result of their membership of the Sub-Group—in a variety of ways in influencing the processing of these issues.

2. LOCAL AUTHORITY, VOLUNTARY AND PRIVATE RESIDENTIAL ESTABLISHMENTS SHOULD BE SUBJECT TO THE SAME SYSTEM OF REGISTRATION AND INSPECTION

This concept is integrated into the National Health Service and Community Care Act 1990, in which the powers of inspection of residential care homes, whether managed by local authority, voluntary or private sector, are set down; the Act did not pass powers of inspection of residential nursing homes to the local authority, although it is anticipated that before a local authority will agree to fund residents in a nursing home, some proof of satisfactory standards of care will be required to be provided by the health authority carrying registering authority.

Local authorities, in general, have accepted their responsibility to register and inspect all residential homes with some rigour and enthusiasm. In order to secure an even-handed approach to the work, the registering and inspection must be done at arms length from the normal line-management responsibilities of local authority staff. To meet this requirement, inspection teams, accountable to the Director of Social Services (or Social Work) have been established; some carry a broad remit to promote quality assurance in all sectors of social service delivery, which may include the management of a comprehensive comments and complaints procedure.

The Sub-Group received the results of a small investigation conducted within the private sector to test how the private sector believed the 'even-handed' requirement of the application of regulations by the local authority to be working. The result of the investigation was inconclusive but there were examples of inconsistent action in individual instances; what could not be substantiated was whether or not the practice would have been different if the situation had arisen in other than the private sector. It is too soon to make firm comment on the general principle, but it is not too soon to comment upon this need for consistency.

Social services in the past have rightly criticised other agencies (such as environmental services) when the change of personnel resulted, on occasions, in substantial change in performance requirements. There must be an agreed standard which has minimal change as a result of personnel involved. There must also be consistency in all sectors not only in the methods of inspecting and reporting, but in the follow-up which takes place to ensure the implementation of any necessary action. The Sub-Group has also kept abreast of the practice guidance issued by the Social Services (and Social Work) Inspectorates, and of their initiatives in monitoring how the new legal requirements are being implemented.

As a secondary function to registration and inspection, the local authority is required to set up an advisory committee which has a duty to monitor the development and practice of the registration and inspection function. There would appear to be less enthusiasm by local authorities to embrace this responsibility. This may arise from the lack of experience of such matters, but it may also be that in the order of priorities this has lesser importance than many of the direct service delivery issues.

In terms of the principle recommended by Wagner, this advisory committee concept is to be welcomed as it provides a further opportunity to monitor even-handedness and choice.

3. THE DEPARTMENT OF HEALTH AND SOCIAL SECURITY (NOW THE DEPARTMENT OF HEALTH) SHOULD DRAW UP NATIONAL GUIDELINES FOR THE INSPECTION OF RESIDENTIAL ESTABLISHMENTS AND SHOULD GIVE EQUAL ATTENTION TO STANDARDS OF ACCOMMODATION, QUALITY OF LIFE, AND THE QUALIFICATIONS OF MANAGEMENT AND STAFF

To date, the Department of Health has declined to issue national guidelines in a prescriptive form, primarily because of the difficulty of ensuring that such guidelines are implemented in a consistent manner throughout the country. The Department, however, has given considerable evidence of their commitment to good practice; this has been achieved by the publication of good practice material and by the funding of research.

In April 1990, the Department of Health (ssi) published 'Homes Are For Living In', which pursued principles such as individuality, dignity and choice, and set them into a pattern of inspection which has been widely accepted as an extremely useful tool. This report has been used as a model by many local authority inspection teams. The Wagner Group commended this publication and all that followed thereafter.

The Department of Health (ssi) then commissioned research by the Department of Social Policy and Social Work at the University of York to assess the feasibility of using a checklist in inspecting the quality of life in old people's homes. This research has been completed and can inform the debate at this time.

The Department of Health (ssi) has produced valuable guidance documents over the years in the 'Caring for Quality' series. These include, under the general title 'Guidance of Standards for Residential Homes', a publication for elderly people, people with a physical disability, and editions for those with mental handicap and mental illness. The first two in the series are a compendium of existing advice to assist in the development of good practice; the latter being new material based on experience.

Another major development by the Department of Health was the substantial funding of the Caring in Homes Initiative programmes, a series of practical projects to test and develop the recommendations of the Wagner Report, to look at standards of care in residential homes, to influence such standards, and to produce material which could be used by practitioners in the future. The Initiative is analysed more fully in Chapter Eight.

It would be reasonable to comment that although national guidelines or procedures, as yet, have not been issued, the result of the Wagner recommendation has been picked up in its spirit and has been thoroughly addressed. The Sub-Group has kept abreast of developments, has often been involved as individuals, and has sought to encourage and facilitate all of the initiatives taken to publicise good practice and how to develop satisfactory standards of quality care.

4. TO ENSURE INDEPENDENCE AND IMPARTIALITY, NO AGENCY SHOULD UNDERTAKE THE INSPECTION OF ITS OWN RESIDENTIAL ESTABLISHMENTS

and

5. AS AN ADJUNCT TO INSPECTIONS, CONSIDERATION SHOULD BE GIVEN TO APPOINTING PANELS OF INDEPENDENT ASSESSORS FROM ALL THREE SECTORS

These concepts appear in the National Health Service and Community Care Act 1990, in the form of 'arms length inspection' and 'advisory committees'. As has already been stated, further time is required to confirm whether or not the spirit of Wagner and of the Act is fulfilled in the mechanisms created. The Sub-Group is heartened by the information available to date and would comment that the aspirations of the Wagner Report may yet be fulfilled.

What is already proved, is that external inspection should not be seen as the only effective system of monitoring and testing standards. Each residential home requires to have a system of internal quality management, a recognised staff development programme, and an effective means of communication between staff, residents, relatives, friends, and the community of which the home is a part. External inspection which then takes place, in addition to such internal structures, will be seen as helpful and constructive, while still retaining the authority of safeguarding the rights of residents, which is the core of all inspection.

The Department of Health consultative document 'Inspecting Social Services' (October 1992) indicates that there is still a strong view that inspection teams should be under the direction of the chief executive of the local authority, rather than have a line-management role to the Director of Social Services.

6. LOCAL AUTHORITIES, VOLUNTARY ORGANISATIONS, AND THE REPRESENTATIVES OF PRIVATE PROPRIETORS

SHOULD PROMOTE SYSTEMS OF SELF-EVALUATION AND PERFORMANCE REVIEW IN ALL RESIDENTIAL ESTABLISHMENTS; NO NEW ESTABLISHMENT SHOULD BE REGISTERED WHICH IS NOT PREPARED TO ADOPT SUCH A SYSTEM

This concept has not found its way into the statute book, but it has established itself in good residential care practice. When the Sub-Group began its work, the subject of quality assurance (in social services terms) was in its infancy; it is now a fully fledged industry and is accepted as legitimate. The Wagner Group is to be commended for its foresight as well as its insight.

In the early days of the Sub-Group, when the work on the checklist concept was at its most active, the Sub-Group agreed that an over-riding principle was that no matter how quality assurance systems are developed, the one undeniable truth is that if standards of care are to be satisfactory to the users, any quality assurance controls must emanate from the beliefs and philosophies which underpin the operation of a particular staff group: any system which 'imposes' a model which is not evident as a part of the staff group *modus operandi* will prove less than satisfactory. With the passing of time, as more and more systems have been developed and publicised, most have confirmed this principle. The Sub-Group remains clear in its view, and reiterates the original thinking.

Inspectors of residential homes, and prior to that, registration officers, are increasingly demanding to see the quality assurance system operation in a home. This is to be encouraged, and it is making such demands of all sectors and reacting in the same manner in similar instances, that evidence of an even-handed approach can be identified.

7. SMALL PRIVATE ESTABLISHMENTS CARING FOR THREE OR FEWER PEOPLE SHOULD BE SUBJECT TO PRELIMINARY VETTING AND TO PERIODIC VISITS; BUT WHERE ONE PROPRIETOR OPERATES A NUMBER OF SUCH HOMES, IN THE SAME NEIGHBOURHOOD, PROVIDING FOR A TOTAL OF FOUR OR MORE RESIDENTS, THEN THE FULL REQUIREMENTS OF THE REGISTERED HOMES ACT SHOULD APPLY

The Registered Homes (Amendment) Act 1991 provides for the registration of homes with fewer than four residents. The fitness of those involved in running the home is the only ground on which registration can be refused. Local authorities have the power, but not the duty, to inspect.

The Department of Health has consulted interested parties on the regulations which should govern these homes. General guidance on the Act has been issued in LAC(91)7 and, following the regulations, further guidance. The Act came into force in April 1993.

The Wagner recommendation, that where one proprietor operates a number of such homes in the same neighbourhood then the full requirements of the Registered Homes Act 1984 should apply, has not been acted upon.

8. RESIDENTIAL ESTABLISHMENTS OPERATING UNDER ROYAL CHARTER SHOULD BE BROUGHT WITHIN THE SCOPE OF THE REGISTERED HOMES ACT

No action has been taken to implement this recommendation. Royal charter was granted in many varied circumstances, and has brought with it an accompanying variety of reactions and results. Some organisations see the royal charter as a means of exclusion from the 'more ordinary' organisation, while others accept it as a tribute but rely little on it for either protection or fund raising. It is suspected that the effort required to amend the legislation in the light of opposition from some quarters is not worth the result. In real terms, the exclusion does not affect large numbers outwith nursing establishments, and many of them are prepared to accept the guidance for residential care, even although they are not required to formally register.

9. RELIGIOUS OR SECULAR COMMUNITIES WHICH CONTINUE TO PROVIDE A HOME FOR MEMBERS WHO HAVE BECOME OLD OR INFIRM SHOULD NOT BE DEEMED TO BE WITHIN THE SCOPE OF THE REGISTERED HOMES ACT

This concept appears to have been fully accepted and the Sub-Group has no evidence of any such community being asked to be subject to the regulations.

10. SERIOUS CONSIDERATION SHOULD BE GIVEN TO A UNIFIED REGISTRATION AND INSPECTION SYSTEM FOR RESIDENTIAL AND NURSING HOMES, TO FACILITATE CONTINUITY OF CARE

This proposal has not been implemented, but the Sub-Group is aware of the work done by the Department of Health to examine examples of good practice. As noted in the comments made on Recommendation 2, operational experience of community care planning agreements between health and local authorities, particularly after April 1993, may yet lead to an application of the concept of joint registration and inspection practice.

As in other aspects of promulgating the recommendations of the Wagner Report, the Department of Health funded research by Rosalind Brooke-Ross into the nature of collaboration between health and social services departments in the task of inspection, of a fact-finding rather than an evaluative basis. It is believed that where there is a will, at local level, to co-operate, mechanisms are developed to make it work. Where co-operation comes about only as a result of policy direction from senior level, the prospect of successful operational experience is greatly reduced. It is also noted that it is easier to put into practice a collaborative approach to inspection, rather than seeking to achieve a joint inspection with one agreed report.

Conclusion

The Sub-Group is able to report that the majority of the recommendations made concerning aspects of quality in residential care have progressed. Some have only moved minimally, in so far as they have been examined closely and a decision taken not to change the *status quo* (as in the instance of royal charter). However, many have moved substantially and have moved ahead the cause of quality options in major strides.

The old question—did he jump or was he pushed?—can be reworded to remind us of the importance of the Wagner Report, and specifically in the field of quality assurance in residential work. *Did they jump or were they pushed?*

Section Two

'A Framework for Quality Assurance in Residential Care'

The Wagner Development Group was among the first to be involved in the issue of how quality assurance could have an impact on the quality of residential care.

The paper produced in 1988 by the Social Care Association and the Association of Directors of Social Services, 'Standard Setting in the Personal Social Services', was referred to the Wagner Development Group, in the hope that the work initiated by those two Associations would be of help to the development of Wagner's aims and objectives. The report was referred to the Quality Assurance Sub-Group which made this its first piece of intensive work. This work resulted in a further report entitled 'Quality Assurance in Residential Care: Devising a Checklist'.

The Sub-Group reported its view that a checklist approach to inspection had some positive attributes if viewed as *a* tool, rather than *the* tool, and if understood within a broader conceptual framework. In other words, the checklist required to be underpinned by principles which required to be understood by the inspector using it. It is not believed that effective inspection can be carried out by using a checklist approach unless the inspector is aware of what is behind the question, comment or observation included in, or required from, the checklist.

Secondly, it was emphasised that to be effective, any quality assurance system must have credibility in the minds of the staff group to whom it is to be applied. The staff group must understand the philosophy which underpins the system, and they must accept it as a credible method of measuring and checking standards of care. Such acceptance and understanding lead to an application of the underpinning principles in care practice in the home.

The report extended the thinking of the earlier SCA/ADSS report, but acknowledged that to translate the work into a full report which would be of long term use in the application of a checklist approach in residential care would require the input of a full-time researcher and writer for about six months.

At the time of reporting to the Development Group, the Sub-Group was aware that the Department of Health had funded research into the feasibility of using a checklist through the Department of Social Policy and Social Work at York University, and had begun to discuss the mechanisms for setting up the Caring in Homes Initiative. The Caring in Homes work has received a wide circulation, together with material to emulate the good practice recorded or developed therein. 'Homes Are For Living In' has been published and widely applied. The Department of Health has issued their series of 'Guidance on Standards for Residential Homes'; many agencies and individuals have developed and promoted material on quality assurance systems; and Newcastle Social Services Department, followed by others, has investigated and pursued the application of British Standard 5750.

As a result of the community care reforms, all care homes are now subject to regular inspection by a local authority inspector. The inspection teams which have grown out of these reforms have enhanced the practice of regular inspection, and there is now a considerable amount of advice and training available.

The Sub-Group was aware of these developments and determined that unless a proper, complete job could be done, little would be achieved by further minimal work at the Sub-Group level. This is still the view of the Sub-Group. The concepts identified in the early work is now integrated into current systems and thinking.

The Sub-Group includes hereafter an adaptation of their work into a framework for quality assurance in residential work, in order that the major principles of the earlier reports can continue to influence the development of good practice.

Mention was made earlier of the application of the British Standard 5750. A British Standard qualification is obtained by seeking registration as a quality assured enterprise from a body certificated by the National Accreditation Council for Certifying Bodies. BS 5750 is a management system which guarantees quality; the application of management systems in this way has long been recognised practice in industry, but only in very recent years has an effort been made to apply the system to social services in general, and to residential care in particular.

The Sub-Group is of the view that all homes should have a quality assurance system and is clear that the existence of such a system does not guarantee quality, since the impact of inter-personal relationships cannot be neatly compartmentalised. The system adopted must be 'owned' by the staff group, and its application should be to direct staff energies towards achieving good care practice.

BS 5750 is a comprehensive system which requires considerable consistent input to maintain certification. It is suggested that the effort to maintain certification detracts from the effort to maintain good care practice, and it is concluded that it is better to adopt a system which is continually directing energies towards good care practice. It is believed that the work done within the Caring in Homes initiative supports this view, and that there are now quality systems available which fulfil this criteria.

Before completing this section, it is necessary to introduce a further issue addressed by the Sub-Group, which has a direct impact on quality in residential settings. This relates to the size of a home, in terms of how many residents can be accommodated, and how the number of residents impacts on quality. It is important to recall that throughout Wagner, Griffiths, and the new legislation, great emphasis is placed on choice. The Sub-Group would suggest that choice includes the size of home in which one chooses to live, and that choice should not be affected by a false argument that only 'small is beautiful'.

The idea that 'small is beautiful' to describe good residential care is often stated as a truism by practitioners and managers. In reality, the question of optimising the quality criteria by deciding on the appropriate number of people who should live in a residential unit has never been satisfactorily resolved. The policy and practice arguments have ranged from issues of privacy to those of choice; creating non-institutional environments to diversity of cost-effectiveness. It appears that research evidence is equally inconclusive.

To a certain extent, the strengths of smaller homes are a weakness of larger homes and *vice versa*. The smaller setting may be characterised as 'homely' and non-institutional, and easier for users and relatives to get involved. However, there may be fewer opportunities to meet other people, to find privacy, and fewer amenities. In contrast, the stereotype of the large establishment may be of formalised systems and regimes which limit choice or involvement rather than an emphasis on available facilities or the benefits of a large staff group. It is evident then, that the criteria of quality is subjective and dependent on preferences.

Efforts to tie the definition to numbers reinforces the view that the question of the size of residential establishments is determined by factors such as the building, its design and location, integration within the local community, the physical facilities it offers. The purpose of the establishment is also important. Nonetheless, it is possible to suggest that there is a notion of optimum size which policy-makers and practitioners to some extent share. Furthermore, in terms of residential care, the numbers vary according to the user group. So that, for example, 'small' for children may be deemed to be four or less, and 'large' above 12; for adult groups, such as people with physical disabilities or learning disabilities, small may be around eight, and large 16 or more; for older people, a small residential unit may be up to 20, and large anything over 30. A further factor is likely to be whether a larger establishment is divided into smaller living groups, especially if these operate on a semi-independent basis.

The aspirations of the Wagner Report offer a series of principles which underpin good quality residential services. The principles of choice, user-involvement, the right to privacy and dignity, respect and individuality are seen as prerequisites to good care. They are not in themselves determined by the size of an establishment or the number of residents who live in one place.

It becomes apparent, therefore, that numbers are only part of the story, along with other factors already mentioned, and in particular the attitude and approach of residential workers. The relationships which exist between those who give and receive care and the leadership offered by managers are likely to be every bit as important, to predicting the quality of life experienced by users. Perhaps we should abandon once and for all any search for a definitive statement on numbers.

There is a widespread acceptance of the need for a framework for quality assurance which focuses on quality of life and standards of management as a means of providing appropriate services for users in residential settings. A core element to quality of life is determined by:

—managing the residential environment to maximise care standards;

—flexible use of regulations and procedures;

—provision of good physical facilities;

—opportunities for users to exercise the principles of rights and unions;

—appropriate attitudes and relationships by staff;

—meeting individual needs.

This section seeks to develop these aspects, in formulating a framework for quality assurance which is capable of having universal application across all sectors and in all establishments providing residential care for adults.

It is acknowledged that this approach to developing a quality assurance system is properly set within the tasks of management.

A Statement of Philosophy

The Wagner Report affirms the valuable role of residential services within the wider spectrum of community care services. In this context it reinforces the importance of the principles of consumer choice and of the positive quality of the residential experience.

Such principles should form the basis of a statement of philosophy which underpins the system of quality assurance. Despite the varied aims and objectives of different residential establishments, these principles reflect a common philosophy within which:

—positive choice is encouraged;

—positive experience is enabled;

—rights are respected and safeguards made explicit;

—continued access to facilities in the community are clarified;

—issues such as respect, dignity, privacy, cultural needs for individuals are explicit within care planning;

—continuity of experience and relationships with relatives and others are maintained.

These principles have been widely applied within the personal social services; they are introduced in 'Home Life', they have been operationalised in 'Homes Are For Living In', and in the SSI Standards documents. They have been tested in practice through the projects in the Caring in Homes Initiative.

Alongside these principles, a range of specific criteria will determine the parameters of any quality assurance system. Legislative factors and local guidelines as standards are also relevant.

Specifying Standards

The need to be explicit in specifying standards appears to be generally agreed within the personal social services. The SSI Standards documents may be seen to have filled an important gap. However, there continues to be confusion around the question of standards, with debate on the need for 'minimum' standards or concentration on 'outcome' standards. The writing of criteria for residential services in ways which are available will undoubtedly be influenced by the increased use of contract specifications.

For the Wagner Development Group, the nature of relationships between users and staff, the ethos and culture, and the management style which prevails within residential establishments irrespective of user group or setting, are essential attributes. It is imperative that this dynamic interactive process is appreciated. Additionally, the use of a regular system of establishment review which is part of a planning and development approach has a valuable potential role, in setting and maintaining high quality standards for residential services.

Developing a Framework for Quality Assurance

A commitment to continued development towards high quality standards is a necessary precursor to a successful quality assurance system. Several features are appropriate in translating commitment into positive action, in ways which improve residential services. The first of these is to determine the need for:

1. clearly defined aims and objectives;

2. a prospectus of the services offered;

3. a written care plan agreed between the user and the establishment;

4. a specified trial period;

5. arrangements for providing advocacy for those requiring assistance with decision-making;

6. a system of regular review for residents;

7. a clear and well publicised complaints procedure;

8. an annual establishment review process with periodic updates, and incorporating the views of users, staff and management;

9. a good practice handbook for all staff;

10. a training plan for the establishment, detailing induction and on-going training, arrangements for staff meetings, supervision and support.

Systematic information gathering should be a regular pattern in the management process. Available information should be used to focus attention in anticipation of review procedures.

Some Practical Considerations

It is apparent from the research work undertaken on the use of checklists that several issues need to be addressed, including standardisation in who completes the forms, what values and criteria they work from, who provides the information, and whether it is possible to check for accuracy.

There is an additional challenge in the involvement of users and others in the collection of audit information.

Diversity of method to quality assurance should reflect the multifaceted aspect of the residential experience. The Department of Health publication 'More Than Meets The Eye' usefully adds to our understanding of the importance of observation skills for those involved in inspection. There are lessons too for managers and practitioners.

The use of a proforma for collecting information, similar to that developed in 'Homes Are For Living In', may provide a useful aide memoire. Typically, sections contain guidance on the methods appropriate to the collecting of information.

Sections generally cover the following areas of examination:

—statistical and administrative information including records, evidence of choice, rights, assessment, review, and keyworking;

—a profile of the users;

—provision of individual packages of care;

—health care arrangements;

—menus, meals and dietary matters;

—premises and facilities, including size of establishment and location;

—staffing;

—support, supervision and training;

—management;

—recording.

All these aspects are important to the development of a framework for quality assurance within a residential establishment. To this end, there should be an annual review which looks back at the previous year and sets an agenda for the forthcoming year. Opportunities should be made to enable discussions with users and their views to be incorporated.

Brief Bibliography

Centre for Policy on Ageing, *Home Life: A Code of Practice for Residential Care*, CPA, 1984
Department of Health/Social Services Inspectorate, *Homes Are For Living In*, HMSO, 1989

Department of Health/Social Services Inspectorate, *Caring for Quality: Guidance on Standards for Residental Homes for Elderly People*, HMSO, 1990

Department of Health, *Inspecting Social Services: A Consultative Document*, DOH, 1992

Social Care Association, *Standard Setting In the Personal Social Services*, SCA, 1988

Wagner Development Group
Aspects of Quality in Residential Care Sub-Group

Ian Baillie
Chairman. Director of Social Work, Church of Scotland Board of Social Responsibility

Charlie Barker
British Association of Social Workers

John Findlay
National Association of Local Government Officers

Lionel Harrison
Observer, Department of Health

Stephen Hey
British Federation of Care Home Proprietors

Des Kelly
Social Care Association

David Lane
Association of Directors of Social Services

Marisa Micallef
National Council for Voluntary Organisations

John Mooney
Observer, Welsh Office

CHAPTER FIVE

Security in Residential Care—
Issues and Concerns

Sub-Group Report

Introduction

The Wagner Report has played a fundamental role in focusing on the needs and rights of residents in residential care homes. One of the Report's aims is to promote good residential care practice which provides residents with as much control over their lives as possible. The recommendations of the Report have provided a framework through which positive choices can be made, both in choosing and living in residential care. The principles and recommendations set out in the Report apply in all residential settings. Residential care, the Report notes, is provided in a wide variety of different types of accommodation for a wide variety of different groups by different organisations. Residential care thus provides both accommodation and care services, and can be distinguished from other forms of provision by the fact that the accommodation and care services are provided in one establishment.

The Report also suggests that the accommodation and care services provided in residential care need to be distinguished, so that people should not be expected to leave their 'place' in order to obtain the care services they need. This link between accommodation and care can create tensions and difficulties in providing residents with the security that the Wagner Report sees as a feature of creating positive choice.

The Sub-Group on security of tenure and residents' rights considered three key questions:

—How can people's accommodation security in residential care be enhanced?

—Can a model or code be promulgated that provides residents with written contracts that offer them security in the accommodation as well as information about the services offered?

—What will be the likely impact of the community care changes on residents' security in residential care?

These questions involve a consideration of both long and short term goals. In the first instance, residents in residential care homes have limited accommodation security. The task of the Sub-Group was to consider how security could be enhanced. In the short term, it was felt that a model or code could be promulgated which aimed to protect residents and offer as much accommodation security or security of tenure as possible within the current administrative and legal framework.

In the longer term, there are a number of proposals which would enhance residents' current insecure position:

—a new legal framework for residents' security of tenure in residential care;

—this would require a new administrative and funding framework, which enables people's accommodation and care needs to be addressed separately;

—this would enable the development of new forms of residential care, which enable accommodation and care needs to be met in a more flexible manner.

Section One

Security in Residential Care

Key considerations

One of the key factors for achieving security in residential care is knowing that the place in which residents live is as much like their own home as possible. In general, in our own homes, we can decide how long we wish to stay and can leave when we choose. As long as we can afford to stay in our present accommodation, this security of tenure provides us with a basic foundation for security in our lives. Yet residents living in residential care homes do not have this basic security of tenure. Generally, when people enter residential care, they give up their housing rights. As a result, residential care is often viewed as the place where care is provided, rather than the place where people also make their home. In the spectrum of accommodation and care services available to vulnerable people, residential care provides little accommodation or housing security.

In housing law (Housing Act 1988), people's legal status as regards their security of tenure moves from a position of substantial security (ie secure or assured tenancies) to virtually no security (bare licences). Residential care provides virtually no security of tenure in law, due to such features as the level of attendance, services or board provided and the extent of sharing accommodation. Security of tenure does not mean the absolute right to stay in accommodation. What it can provide, however, is a legal framework and a set of conditions which determine when and under what defined circumstances a person has to leave. It also provides a method by which people can question or confirm their position. Without a change in legislation, any rights to some element of accommodation security in residential care depends on the contract (written or verbal) determined between the resident and the provider of the home on payment of the charge for the accommodation and services.

A Contract for Accommodation and Services

The provision of a written contract for accommodation and services is a key recommendation of the Wagner Report. This recommendation provides the opportunity not only to ensure that residents are aware of the services available, but it can provide a mechanism, in the short term, by which the security of residents in residential care could be enhanced. At present, there is no legal right to a written contract although, under the Registered Homes Act 1984, many registration authorities do expect a written contract or statement to be provided. What is, however, essential in developing written contracts is the need to ensure that contracts cover the main areas of concern and interest for residents and providers, in relation to both the accommodation and the care services provided in residential care.

There are already examples of good practice in the provision of written contracts in residential care which offer simple explanations of residents' rights and responsibilities, and offer an explanation of residents' accommodation security. There are also examples of poor practice which place unexplained restrictions on residents' freedom or lifestyle, and offer a limited explanation of their accommodation position. Since the contract can play a key role in defining the relationship between residents and providers, the promulgation of good practice in this field is essential. At present, as with accommodation security, residents have few rights to receive specific statements about their residential establishment.

What are the Impediments to Providing more Accommodation Security in Residential Care?

From the provider's point of view, there are limitations to offering security of tenure, due to the fact that residential care offers both accommodation and care services. For a number of reasons, providers resist an extension of security of tenure. The primary concern is the fact that residents' care needs change over time. There is also a concern about the problems created by a 'disruptive' resident in a residential community. Factors which create these concerns include the impact of the registration system which distinguishes between care for residents in homes and the problem of residents moving in rehabilitative schemes when they no longer need the level of care provided.

Registration

One solution recommended by the Wagner Report is to offer a unified registration system for both residential and nursing homes. This could allow greater flexibility for providers by enabling them to offer both short and longer term extra care themselves, without having to alter their registration standards. The new inspection units under the NHS and Community Care Act—with the greater emphasis on quality of life—should serve to focus yet again on the known difficulties of the present system. A unified system providing flexible and wide-ranging registration standards with guidance from the centre could create a climate whereby providers can feel more comfortable, with greater accommodation security for residents.

Domiciliary Extra Care

People living in residential care need to have the same access to domiciliary health and social services as people living in the community. In theory this is the case but in practice there are many instances of a lack of provision, given limited resources in the public sector, for those living in residential care. For those who can afford it, buying in extra services can also create problems with the dual registration system. It is the provider who is often left to resolve increasing care needs themselves, and this can often mean the only solution is to move a resident to an alternative establishment. The new assessment and care management proposals under the NHS and Community Care Act could create a situation where care needs are reassessed by a care manager and appropriate 'client centred' care packages delivered, wherever people live. If the residential accommodation is also more secure, and such assessments consider both accommodation and care needs, a resident should only be expected to move if and when it is the sensible and acceptable solution to that person (or their advocate in the case of the most vulnerable).

Moving

Some providers are offering shorter stay accommodation for vulnerable groups to prepare them for independent living. Their concerns about offering more accommodation security are related to the need to be able to move people on to more independent settings, when the special support and care provided in that accommodation is no longer required. However, in the case of existing secure or assured tenancies, one of the grounds for possession is that a person no longer requires the 'social services or special facility' provided in the accommodation. In this case reasonable and suitable accommodation must be provided. Offering more security with specific grounds for asking people to leave such as this one, would allow far more housing rights than the present position. Of course, the concern of this group of providers is broader too, and relates to the lack of accommodation for 'move on'. This is a wider issue, also recognised by the Wagner Report.

Disruptive Residents

Providers are concerned about disruptive and violent behaviour, which can be acute in residential care where people share living arrangements. Any improvement in security of tenure for residents in residential care would require a proper and expedient means of dealing with such behaviour which ensured that the provider, often acting on behalf of other residents, was able to resolve the difficulties but also that the disruptive resident's needs and rights were also considered. The National Federation of Housing Associations drafted a clause in their model agreement which meets this issue, and should provide some comfort to providers concerned about meeting the needs of the residential community.

A Move to Greater Security?

Security of tenure will not mean that residents cannot be asked to move in certain circumstances. A framework, which provides residents with a clearer notion of their rights and responsibilities as far as their accommodation is concerned, needs to highlight notice periods and specified grounds for possession which reflect the particular features of residential care, whilst enhancing residents' security.

Can a Resident's Contract for Accommodation and Services be Promulgated?

The Sub-Group, in developing the Wagner recommendation on contracts by working on a model contract or agreement, had as one of its aims the enhancement of residents' security and other rights in residential care. Existing examples of good practice in this field were drawn upon. The starting point was to offer a code or model to be used in all sectors, which offered residents in residential care as much security as possible, whilst recognising some of the impediments to providing full security in the shorter term.

Such a code is presented in Section 2. However the mechanism for establishing residents' rights to such a contract needs to be developed. There are also a number of essential considerations for drawing up written contracts. Firstly, whilst contracts need to be as unrestrictive as possible, it is accepted that the responsibilities of providers, through registration conditions for example, and the fact of community living and shared accommodation, will mean restrictions may need to be placed on residents' rights. What is essential, however, is that contracts include an explanation where any restrictions are imposed and such restrictions should not be unreasonable. Secondly, an acceptable and proper procedure needs to be clarified where residents, due to vulnerability or incapacity, are unable to enter into a contract. The effective use of advocates or appointees needs to be clarified in developing the code.

There are a number of mechanisms through which a written contract with specified terms could be enhanced. Firstly, the existing registration system can be used not only to promote further the use of written contracts, but also to set out the particular terms that ought to be covered. The new inspection units with general advice from the centre, provide an opportunity to consider this mechanism for improving good practice. Secondly, the contracting proposals for residential care services under community care legislation, delayed until 1993, provide for a greater role for local authorities. They ensure that a proper written agreement or accommodation and services is provided for residents where they are contracting residential services. Thirdly, there could be a new legal framework established whereby all residents in residential care homes are entitled, by law, to a written contract in a specified form. These options can only be developed if a code or model can be developed, and is acceptable and workable for all residential settings.

Impact of Community Care Changes on Residents' Security in Residential Care

A written statement about accommodation and services can only be described as a contract if a financial transaction is undertaken by the parties to the contract. Without this, there may be doubts about the creation of a proper contract in law. The community care proposals on local authorities contracting services, including residential care, lead to some concern about how a contract between a resident and the provider of the residential services can be facilitated. The proposals on contracting determine that it is the local authority who will pay the provider for the residential place, although there is some provision within the legislation to allow residents to pay homes directly for their accommodation, but not their care costs.

Much of the discussion about contracting arrangements under the new community care system has focused on the contracts to be determined between the local authority and the provider. In order to maintain and promote the rights and needs of residents as set out in the Wagner Report, it is necessary to consider the three way relationship (established between resident, provider and local authority). It is also important to ensure that residents are entitled to a written statement of their rights and responsibilities in residential care. The resident thus needs to be at the centre of the contract relationship. Government, in terms of advice, and local authorities will have a key role to play in developing this issue.

Further consideration of the effects of these new proposals on residents' rights in residential care will be required if the recommendations of the Wagner Report on positive choice are to be met.

Section Two

Code for a Contract

This is a reduced version of the full text, which is available separately.

Guidance Notes

Why Is a Code for a Contract Needed?

A residential care home provides a person with a home as well as personal care. Residents living in such homes have very few clearly defined legal rights. Rules and regulations of the home may leave residents with little control over their daily activities and, in some cases, lead to the denial of basic freedoms.

The first step to giving basic rights to residents in this situation, is to ensure that each resident has a formal written contract. A contract is intended to ensure that residents are properly informed of their rights and responsibilities when they move into a home and this Code sets a framework for drawing up such a contract.

The aim of the Code is to set out good practice in drawing up contract terms for residents living in residential care homes, within the current legal and administrative framework.

Who Will Use the Code?

The Code is intended as a set of guiding principles for providers to use in drawing up written contractual agreements with residents. The Code is primarily intended for residential care schemes which are either local authority Part III accommodation or have to conform to the requirements of the Registered Homes Act 1984, including small homes. The Code is therefore aimed at providers in the local authority, private, voluntary and housing association sectors. Purchasers may find the code useful, and may wish to adopt some of its principles in drawing up service specifications. Prospective residents, or their representatives, may wish to use the Code in making an assessment of a home's contract.

The Code should apply to all the different adult categories contained in the Registered Homes Act 1984, who live in residential care schemes, including elderly people, people with mental health problems, people with learning difficulties, people with physical disabilities and people with drug and alcohol problems. The Code should also apply to people within these categories with particular needs, for instance black people and ethnic minorities, people with AIDS or HIV and homeless people.

What Is a Contract?

A contract is an agreement between two or more parties, supported by a consideration, with the intention of creating a legal relationship. A consideration is anything of material value which is offered by one party in exchange for a consideration from the other party, for instance exchange of accommodation for rent. Contracts for residential care homes can, therefore, apply where a resident pays the home a fee for accommodation and related services. This could apply where the resident was only paying some of the fee, with the rest coming from elsewhere.

There are circumstances where the fee is not paid to the home by the resident, and is either paid to the home by a person acting on behalf of the resident, or paid by the local authority where the resident is fully 'sponsored'. In these circumstances the home could either issue a contract to the resident as if it were a legal agreement, or enter into a joint contract with the resident and fee payer. Where residents are mentally incapacitated, for instance through the effects of dementia, it may be necessary for the contract to be signed by a relative, or an appointee, or for an advocate to represent the resident. Where a contract is signed by another party on behalf of the resident, legal advice may have to be sought on the status of the contract. This is a difficult and problematic area, which will need more active work in the future.

Whatever is written into a contract, it cannot remove residents' statutory rights. Provisions contained in legislation such as the Race Relations Act 1976 and the Sex Discrimination Act 1975 provide protection for residents, not only against discrimination by managers or owners, but also against discrimination perpetuated by other residents. More specific legislation such as the Unfair Contract Terms Act 1977 also applies.

Use of the Code

The Code aims to be used for drawing up contracts under many different circumstances. A significant number of residents living in residential care homes are private payers and responsible for their own fees. These residents should have individual contracts with the provider. Residents on low incomes living in independent sector residential care homes are eligible for a higher rate of DSS income support to meet their accommodation and care costs. These residents should have individual contracts with the provider. The contracts would be valid even if income support is paid direct.

Under the new community care arrangements, there is a change from the system of DSS funding of the independent sector which supports housing and care costs together, to a system which supports housing and care costs separately. Local authorities will assess individual's care needs and enter into contractual arrangements with providers of residential care, to purchase places for people needing this type of care. The local authority contract will define what services it wants for the individual. At the same time it would be good practice for providers to define their relationship with the users through a separate contract.

Housing associations are required to have a legal relationship with their residents/tenants. This has to be in the form of a written agreement in exchange for a fee or rent. The NHS and Community Care Act 1990 enables such an arrangement to take place and residents can pay providers the element of the charge which would have been paid to local authorities to offset the full costs of the placement.

The Code

The Code is structured into three parts and makes a distinction between: accommodation and services, operational policies, and care and support services. These three elements should together form the contract between the home and the resident.

Accommodation and Services This part should form the main document for the contract and is known as the occupancy agreement. The Code sets out main principles for the terms of occupancy and the rights of residents to accommodation and related services. This part of the contract should also make reference to the parts covering the operational policies and the care and support services.

Operational Policies

The second part of the contract should include all the policies and procedures for running the home. This part can either be appended to the main document, or contained in a separate residents' handbook.

Care and Support Services

This part of the contract should include the philosophy of care of the home, and the resident's individual care plan. This part of the contract may be subject to regular review to take account of the changing care needs of individual residents.

Accommodation and Services

People living in residential care homes have no security of tenure. Residential care homes providers should ensure that residents have a written occupancy agreement, as part of an overall contract, which provides them with a number of contractual rights and informs them of their obligations.

Good Practice

Written Agreement

Occupancy agreements should always be in writing

Notice   The period of notice (by resident and provider) should not be less than four weeks

Grounds for Termination   There should be specific grounds for termination of the contract

Obligations of the Resident   The obligations of the resident should be clearly spelt out

Payment of Charges/Fees   The details of the payment of charges/fees for accommodation, related services and care should be clearly identified

Occupancy   The provider should allow the resident to occupy his or her room without interruption or interference and receive the services detailed in the contract

Maintenance and Repair   Providers should keep their homes properly maintained and repaired

Complaints   The resident should have the right to make complaints about the services provided

Equal Opportunities   Providers should have a clear equal opportunities statement

Consultation   Residents should have a right to be consulted before changes are made to the provider's policies and practices which may have a substantial effect on the resident

Information   Residents should have a right to information on the operational policies of the home.

The legal position of residents' tenure and statutory rights relating to residential accommodation is largely defined by the Housing Act 1988. Residents living in residential care homes are most likely to be licensees, as opposed to tenants. A licence is merely permission to occupy granted to an individual and is personal to that individual and cannot be passed on. A tenant has a considerable number of statutory rights and the extent of these rights depends upon the type of tenancy.

Licensees have no security of tenure and there are no legal grounds which could limit the action of providers of residential care homes. The Housing Act 1988 has, however, strengthened the Protection from Eviction Act 1977 to give private sector tenants and licensees greater protection from harassment and illegal eviction, although public sector, charitable or registered housing association licensees have been 'excluded' from these provisions.

Despite the fact that residents living in residential care homes have few legal rights, it is good practice that they should have a number of contractual rights written into their occupancy agreement. The key features of ensuring that residents have some security of tenure involves issues such as defining the basis on which people can be asked to leave, how much notice they are given and explaining their rights to occupy the home. These aspects and other contractual rights are discussed in detail in the full text of the Code.

Operational Policies

The operational policies of the home need to be clearly set out, so that both the residents and providers are clear about how the home is run. Some of the policies outlined below should be adapted to the particular needs of the residents.

Good Practice

User Involvement	The home should include residents in any decisions which affect their lives
Catering	There should be a clear explanation about the catering arrangements
Visitors	There should be a clear policy on visitors
House Rules	If there are any house rules, they should be clearly stated

Complaints Procedure	There should be a formal complaints procedure, which should be simple, clear and have a precise time limit for completion
Equal Opportunities Policy	There should be a written policy which covers all aspects of the services provided
Harassment Policy	There should be a clear written statement of policy on harassment
Arrears Policy	Providers should have a clear arrears policy which minimises the possibility of eviction
Repairs and Maintenance Procedures	There should be clear procedures on repairs and maintenance
Health and Safety Policies	The health and safety policies of the home should not restrict residents' choices, except where reasonable to ensure the safety of other residents and the home
Drugs and Medicine Policy	The home should have a clear written drugs and medicine policy
Policy for Restraint	Restraint should only be used if it is necessary for protection.

There needs to be a document explaining how each residential care home is run and the facilities and services available. This document can either form a second part of the contract or stand alone as a residents' handbook. In either case the accommodation agreement would need to make references to the document, which would go into greater detail on particular policies. This document, or handbook, would be a key source of information for potential residents or local authorities choosing a home, as well as providing existing residents with clear policies and procedures.

The Registered Homes Act 1984, and related regulations, require local authorities to ensure that homes meet both minimum physical standards, as well as good operational standards. Local registration officers are increasingly requiring homes to have clear written policies and procedures on a number of issues.

In terms of residents' rights the regulations require that residents' wishes and feelings should be taken into account. The regulations also place an obligation on the registered person to provide each resident with a written statement of the complaints procedure, including details of how to complain directly to the registration authority.

These policies and procedures would need to be translated for people living in the home whose first language is not English. Furthermore, the home needs to ensure that the policies and procedures take account of the particular needs of black people and ethnic minorities. Further discussion of 'good practice' is contained in the full text of the Code.

Care and Support Services

Residents living in residential care homes should have as much control and choice as possible. A contract should outline the principles on which the care and support services are based and how they can be best achieved. The Department of Health publication 'Homes Are For Living In' sets out a useful framework and we have used this as a starting point.

Good Practice

Privacy	Residents should have the right to privacy whenever they want it
Dignity	Residents' self-respect should be safe-guarded and their personal needs respected
Independence	Residents should be able to retain as much independence as possible, including the right to take personal risks
Choice	Residents should be free to make their own decisions
Rights	The rights of residents to basic freedoms should be safe-guarded

Fulfilment Residents should be enabled to achieve their potential capacity—physical, intellectual, emotional and social.

The care and support services in a residential care home can only be successful if they are informed by a clear set of aims and common values. A contract should reflect these aims and values, so that residents are informed about the principles of the care services provided. Individual care plans are a means of implementing the principles of care within a home and tailoring them to the specific needs of individuals.

Translating these care and support principles into practice involves taking account of individual resident's particular needs and respecting their individuality. Drawing up individual care plans in consultation with residents and, where appropriate, their relatives or an advocate, enables a clear statement to be made about what the resident can expect on a day-to-day basis and what the home should provide. Care plans should be reviewed on a regular basis to take account of the fact that individuals' needs change. The contract with the resident should include their individual care plans to ensure the needs of the individual are a central part of the contract. Where an individual's care plan changes, this part of the contract can be amended without having to change the whole document. The full text of the Code elaborates further on 'good practice' in this area.

Brief Bibliography

Department of Health/Social Services Inspectorate, *Purchase of Service: Practical Guidance and Practice Material for Social Services*, HMSO, 1991

National Federation of Housing Authorities, *Guide for Legal Status of Residents Living in Shared Housing Schemes*, NFHA, 1988

National Federation of Housing Authorities, *The 1988 Housing Act*, NFHA, 1990

National Federation of Housing Authorities, *Licence Agreement and Assured Tenancy Agreement for Shared Housing*, NFHA, 1992

Wagner Development Group
Security of Tenure and Residents' Rights Sub-Group

Ian Baillie
Director of Social Work, Church of Scotland Board of Social Responsibility

Chris Beddoe
Consultant, Chris Beddoe & Associates

Stephen Campbell
Association of County Councils

James Churchill
Association for Residential Care

David Lane
Association of Directors of Social Services

Barbara Meredith
National Council for Voluntary Organisations

Marisa Micallef
Chairman. National Council for Voluntary Organisations

Cliff Prior
Stonham Housing Association

Guy Robertson
Association of Metropolitan Authorities

David Wolverson
Anchor Housing Association

Past Members

Mike Ashley
Association of District Councils

Brian Jones
Association of Metropolitan Authorities

Jane Minter
National Council for Voluntary Organisations (formerly Chairman)

Nick Moore
Policy Studies Institute

Antony Pittaccio
European Confederation of Care Home Owners

Sheila Scott
National Care Homes Association

CHAPTER SIX

Black Perspectives on Residential Care
Sub-Group Report

Introduction

The Wagner Reports like many such reports before it, failed to address the crucial issue of black people's rights to a 'positive choice'. As a result, the Wagner Development Group requested the Race Equality Unit (REU) to undertake a piece of work to examine residential care from a black perspective. The REU subsequently commissioned this work through the establishment of a Black Perspectives group, which formed a Sub-Group of the Wagner Development Group. The Black Perspectives Sub-Group accordingly undertook a study, the results of which were published in full by NISW in 1992 as 'A Home From Home'. The text which follows here summarises the larger lines of the study, emphasising the crucial issues—for both black and white people.

It is a truism that social services and related mainstream agencies have not adequately fulfilled their responsibilities in providing sensitive social care to black families and their communities. In general, the nature of services provided (or available) has either exacerbated the social problems experienced by black families with controlling and disempowering outcomes, or has failed to respond to their social needs; and the manner in which the services have been planned and resourced has left the black community at the periphery of the service provision at best, or outside the service agencies at worst.

For black communities, residential care has not only been unequal and inappropriate, but inaccessible and unavailable as well. On the one hand, those members of the black community who have received mainstream residential care have experienced prejudice and racism which has denied them their cultural reality, racial pride, self-dignity and black identity. On the other hand, myths and stereotypes of black families such as 'they look after their own', 'residential care is not part of their culture', have worked against the interests and welfare of their members in need of residential care.

In the past few years, the philosophy and quality of residential care has gone through critical evaluation out of which has emerged a push for change not least as a consequence of the Wagner Report. There is now greater advocacy for transforming residential care from institutionalised services to personal services, where residents can live a life with choice, options, dignity and esteem, not forgetting a sense of belonging. This is based on a firm belief that residential care should not be a dumping resort or a poor option for users and that the standard of care must be maximised to enhance the quality of residential life. It cannot be stressed enough that this transformation must take account of the black experience, as no other experience has exposed the shortcomings of residential care so acutely and painfully.

There is considerable evidence which demonstrates not only that black people are not receiving the care to which they are entitled, but also that while being under-represented in the welfare provision of social work, they are over-represented in the controlling aspects of social work. Surveys have indicated that the view black people have of social services departments is that they fail to offer relevant services, and as a consequence are used as a last resort only.

At a policy and planning level, the situation provides little scope for optimism. The disproportionate number of black children and black persons with mental illness in residential care, and little or no presence of black elders, disabled and black persons with learning difficulties in residential care are not accidental. There is a direct connection between the over-representation of certain members of black communities in residential settings, and control and under-representation of other members of black communities and welfare. Any further debates on black people and residential care need to acknowledge this, understand it within the context of racist oppression and deal with it.

This scenario of lack of appropriate services, coupled with the experiences of black people and their families in accommodation geared to the needs of white people (and therefore by definition the exclusion of black people) has led to black people organising and securing appropriate care in residential accommodation geared specifically to meet their needs. This care has predominately taken the form of black-led voluntary and private organisations, although there are also some examples of provision in the statutory sector.

Section One

The Experience of Black Residential Projects

The aims of the study carried out by the Black Perspectives Sub-Group were:

1. To explore projects which are established specifically to provide residential care to black people.

2. To identify and develop models of good practice in residential care for black communities from material thus obtained.

3. To highlight areas of work for further research and development.

The primary purpose was to identify ways and approaches that would be effective and useful for moving forward in enabling residential care to be delivered in a manner which is relevant and appropriate to black people, their families and communities. The methodology employed to collate information reflected the conviction that black projects provide examples of good practice, which is informed by their experience of the provision of appropriate services to black communities. The study explored the work of eight residential establishments. The projects which agreed to participate provide a range of services:

—to children;

—to young mothers;

—to adolescents;

—to elderly people.

The findings of the study which follow are organised within the context of practice and service issues, using headings for ease of reference and not in any order of priority.

1. ADVANTAGES OF BLACK LEADERSHIP IN PROVIDING RESIDENTIAL AND PERSONAL CARE

The emergence of black voluntary organisations providing residential care has not been in a vacuum. While such residential provisions have been the outcomes of active responses to establish alternative services in the absence of mainstream services, more importantly black-led residential care has been rooted in the black history and tradition of care. The philosophy of looking after the vulnerable members of communities and taking care of family and community members is right at the heart of black culture and the way of life. Black-led residential care is a continuation of the caring tradition and manifestation of the caring philosophy. While the failure of (white) residential establishments in providing appropriate care to black people is part of this scenario, it is not the entirety. Black people are not only reacting to white failings, but are creative, skilful and able to identify and meet their own needs, and it must be acknowledged that the blockages of white control and racism have sought to prevent them from doing so.

A clear philosophy underpinned most of the projects involved in the study. This clarity encompassed an agreement of needs which is based on the acknowledgment, understanding and experience of racism and its effects. It is important to highlight here some differences between the one establishment that was not black-led and the other projects. In providing a service to both black and white residents, while they had a clear philosophy, this did not integrate black people's experience of racism. The realisation that there was a need for appropriate care for black elders was precipitated through the admission of an Asian Moslem elder to the home. This is in marked contrast to the black-led homes in the study, which were based on an understanding of racism as the starting point of service provision, as opposed to a process which was underpinned by lack of services—one is a proactive process and the other is reactive. In the latter case, the situation then developed of the issues of racism having to be dealt with as an afterthought, not as integral to the process of change. The process of change focused not on the black experience, but on the white perception of the black experience which was founded on notions of exotic culture and language. Staff therefore had to be convinced, trained and cajoled into an understanding of racism and its effects, whereas in black-led homes, this was the starting point, and therefore the understanding ipso facto existed. This fundamental philosophical base was the keystone on which meeting the needs of black residents was built and was reflected in the experiences of both children and adults in black-led homes, where they did not have to convince carers of the importance of their cultural traditions. In relation to children, developing a sense of self-worth, being able to locate their place in the community, and learning to cope with matters which affect them as black children were identified as critical. This included the development of pride in who they were and a feeling of ease with themselves. This facilitated their return to black families and the black community with less disruption and a greater ability to deal with the experience of care. This contrasts sharply with the experiences of black children in white-led homes.

A fundamental issue affecting practice here is the underlying acknowledgement and acceptance the homes had that all black children are part of the black community. This aspect guided all decisions and actions. The marked difference here is the debate that white workers engage in when attempting to decide where the child belongs, and therefore they develop practice which is based on under-estimating or misunderstanding the need for belonging and cultural and racial identity.

This philosophy applied to all black children, including those with one parent who was white. For these children, in particular, it provided the necessary base line for helping them to work through problems relating to identity confusion, problems related to negative feelings about being black and poor self-images, and also in helping them to develop the strengths to deal with racism in a society which would always view them as black. The value of this philosophical base is that in valuing the black heritage of these children, their white heritage and parentage was not negated. It is extremely difficult within a report like this to encapsulate the importance of the values that are intrinsic to such a philosophy and this particular aspect of the study has left us without doubt that care for all black children can never meet their needs, unless it incorporates care by black adults.

Elders found reassurance and comfort in being with others from a similar background. The common bond existed of originating from Africa or the Indian subcontinent, but with considerable cultural and life experience difference between islands in the Caribbean or differences between Gujerati and Punjabi Asian people. These differences were not a source of conflict and provided a reason for finding out about each other, sharing information, learning and establishing commonalities, without the negative effects of racism. It gave elders a sense of being valued and wanted in a society which is generally hostile to them. Matters of racism and cultural traditions were taken as read, and allowed people to progress with other issues, without these becoming the only focus of attention. Essentially the approach and philosophy of black-led homes can be described as holistic, an approach which not only recognises and seeks to care for the whole person, responding to body, mind and spirit, but also places that individual within the context of their family, and their community.

Another major aspect of black leadership in homes is the 'community approach'. This recognises and understands the needs of the community, and adopts a flexible approach to the needs of both the community and the individual as they arise. The reverse could be said to be true of white-led organisations, which establish 'rules' (in the form of assessment procedures etc) and expect individuals and communities to fit into their regulations, not vice-versa. Such an approach is not only an indication of their flexibility, but also of their creativity and ability to develop services and respond to a range of needs despite the constraints of tight budgets, and the restrictions of the local authority.

A community approach incorporating these characteristics should not be confused with 'disorganisation', or 'unprofessionalism', labels which are often attached to black-led projects. Structures and systems clearly exist and work in such projects, but these do not function to restrict initiative, rather to accommodate it. The shared experience of both staff and users ensures an environment where trust and confidence can be established. For example, experiences of past or current racism do not have to be explained in 'rational', ie unemotional terms, but can be shared or explored in an environment which is empathic and rational, rather than judgmental or collusive. Anger can be freely displayed, without requiring justification or explanation. At a broader level, there appeared to be more expression of feeling than is experienced in white-led children's homes. An example is the expression of anger, which was regarded as positive and healthy whether by staff or residents. The size of establishment clearly has an effect on the service offered. Black projects tend to be smaller: this is not by accident, but rather by design. Local authority service users have encountered a number of difficulties which are a result of being housed in large, inflexible institutions. Black projects have sought to avoid these obstacles.

Cultural identity, encompassing different values, traditions, linguistic, artistic and religious attributes is none the less very important in providing appropriate care for people; but what the study revealed is that this is achieved not by having 'Bob Marley' pictures on the wall or by having curry on the menu, but through a holistic approach which is evident in the feel and smell of the establishment, and the sense of belonging and peace which is created by black people by their presence. Indeed, to the Sub-Group, the physical environment of the home, eg books, ornaments etc, seemed of less importance than they had expected. They found that in their experience of white-led homes, racial and cultural identity, although expressed visually in some places, was, in effect, used to divert attention away from the fundamental issue of racism that creates the very conditions in which the culture of some groups is devalued. It also led to an over-reliance on cultural explanations to explain human behaviour or problems. This is the very backbone of multi-culturalism, the shibboleth of a patronising liberalism that encourages one to acknowledge cultures of so-called ethnic minorities whilst leaving intact the racism of the dominant white majority. Black staff within the project establishments understood this issue, and central to their experiences was therefore an understanding of what identity means and the knowledge that for black people, this does not separate out from being black. This is in marked contrast to white workers who grapple unsuccessfully with the concept, and conclude that for a child or elderly person being black is an 'additional need' to be met, rather than the context in which their needs should be met. Such muddled thinking leads to muddled practice, and black people in need of care suffer as a consequence.

2. PRACTICAL CARE

The components which contribute towards appropriate care for black people should not be viewed in isolation from each other, but rather part of a whole process of care.

Languge was viewed as a major issue in terms of the spoken language (ie English, Gujerati etc) and also the use of language, and the language environment of the organisation. It was found to be essential that workers and residents were able to relate orally, both in terms of worker to resident, and also resident to resident. Language is not only about the actual spoken word, but also about the meaning attributed to the use of particular words within a cultural and experiential framework. The commonality of understanding in relation to these goes some way to ensuring that people feel valued. The issue of language is viewed by the Sub-Group as an essential feature of good care which provides a common bond between staff and residents and for elders in particular, has the effect of lessening isolation and increasing feelings of importance. Even for children whose language was English, the Sub-Group found 'Black English' and patios served a similar function. Language is more than communication: crucial though 'good' communication is in providing 'good' care, it is also about freedom of expression, release of emotions, cultural identity and shared values.

The language environment within a home or day-centre should fulfil the resident's right to be understood without a constant battle to be understood, or without having to justify the need/importance of this to white workers. The study highlighted the fact that where the language environment is appropriate, stress and anxiety levels are considerably reduced.

In one home providing care for people from several linguistic backgrounds, the issue of a resident speaking a language which staff were unable to understand arose. In this case, access to a 24 hour interpreter was seen as vital, alongside regular sessions, both for the user and their family. Similarly, the translation of written material is important. Where people are not literate even in their own language it is still important that information is translated: it demonstrates respect and accords dignity, and most people can find someone who can read something to them.

Access to and use of natural medicine such as herbalism was regarded particularly by elders as being important to their sense of well being. Some of the homes in the study were open to exploring the possibility of alternative medicine, and often tips for 'cures' were picked up by staff through contact with members of the community. The greatest source of knowledge was from the elders themselves who had a wealth of tradition and expertise around health care. This is very different from the experience of elderly people in white-led homes where the only experts are the GPs and residents are not expected to contribute to their own health care. The value of having workers who can not only be receptive to the possibility of using traditional medicines but will also actively seek and utilise the wisdom of other black people is very clear. One Asian woman, during an interview, turned to a member of staff to remind him that he must remember to liquidise her Kerala. He reassured her that he had not forgotten and understood that this was not merely an eating fad, but that the liquid from this vegetable was a natural method through which she controlled her diabetes.

There was also an understanding by most of the staff that black people are particularly affected by certain health conditions, eg thelasaemia, sickle cell anaemia, diabetes and high blood pressure etc and that the home environment needs to be a place in which stress and anxiety are reduced, thereby helping to contribute to the prevention and treatment of these conditions. Residents also seemed well aware of this and home was viewed as a kind of haven where one would not experience the stress of racism that occurs outside.

With young people, staff assumed an educative role and, in some homes, organised sessions on sickle cell and other health related issues.

Regular meetings of residents are a mechanism for ensuring the integral involvement of residents in decisions taken in the establishments. It is important that meetings are 'free-flowing', not merely a forum for endorsing decisions already made by management of the home.

Food was viewed by all homes as a crucial factor in creating an atmosphere of comfort and belonging:

No one turns up their noses at the smell of my food.

The range of different foods provided by the establishments which the Sub-Group visited was surprising. Each establishment provided a variety which gave residents real choice in their individual food preferences. In some homes, particularly those catering for younger people, they were encouraged to cook their own food. This not only develops survival skills, but also contributes to a sense of control over an important aspect of life. Children were invited to widen their experience by trying food which they may not have experienced thus far. Elders on the other hand were able to share their culinary expertise with staff by teaching them about the preparation of food. This provided an important role for elders, and in one establishment they had been involved in the recruitment of the cooks and were then helping to train them up . As one man said, 'at first the food wasn't so good, but we've been teaching them and it is getting better, although it's not like my mother's cooking'. The elders took a real pride in their knowledge of cooking, and felt respected in that their views were sought and contributed to improving the quality of care for everyone. Knowing who is preparing the food is as important as having the right type of food.

Food is not just about 'eating' at meal times but is a source for engaging in social relationships. Residents conveyed the importance of not feeling 'odd' or being an object of curiosity because they were eating their 'own' food.

The involvement of family was viewed as crucial, not only in terms of assisting staff to make the 'right' decisions, but also creating an atmosphere which made them feel welcome. Elders had a strong sense of mutual caring, not only in relation to other residents, but also to workers and their families. Some elders had a strong feeling that they had been let down by their families, and therefore not only in many cases had to adjust psychologically to not returning 'home', but also to the inevitability that they will not live the remaining years of their lives with their families.

The elders have nevertheless coped with their changing circumstances and expectations, and are still able to be positive about their families and themselves. Some had strong links with their families, whilst some did not. In some cases the mutual feeling of rejection formed a common bond between the elders. In white homes the feeling of rejection is usually not reduced but often increased to 'being dumped'.

In most cases, the families of staff members at these homes were also in some way involved in the running of the home.

A shared faith and the practice of religion was supported and encouraged. A strong sense of spirituality prevailed in some homes, with joint worship, and a sharing of spiritual experience, eg through singing.

3. STAFFING

The study demonstrated clearly that the type of care provided depends very much on the type of management and staff that are employed. Staffing also has a bearing on the impression that the community has of the home. The importance of appropriate staffing cannot therefore be overemphasised.

The under-resourcing of the homes in the study resulted in limited formal staff development and training. The release of staff has cost implications in terms of cover for the home when the staff are away on training. This situation led to the restriction of opportunities for staff in seeking professional training and qualifications. However, it also meant that managers were innovative and creative in setting up training programmes and sharing skills and expertise through networks. The use of independent black trainers and consultants has developed to provide in-house training but this is limited to a few projects. Where available, such training provides a wider perspective and ensures that workers are informed of changes in legislation, the development of practice, as well as generating support networks and forums for workers to experiment and be challenged in.

Evidence from the projects suggests that whereas key worker and counsellor systems occur in children's establishments, this is not the case in those for elders. The principle of key workers is important, but is not the only system which can be employed. It cannot be disputed that clear care plans are good practice and should extend to all residents, regardless of which 'client group' they are perceived as belonging to.

Care plans should be drawn up with residents and if appropriate their families or friends. They provide an opportunity for people to say what help they need in caring for themselves and to negotiate how this help should be given. The process allows residents to share with staff the issues that are important to them and is a means by which they can maintain some control over their own lives. Within the study, several projects used care plans. These did not have race and culture as aspects to be considered but as central to the care of the person; so that the questions became (for example) not whether a child's contact with a grandma in Jamaica was important, but how that contact should be maintained. This example demonstrates the way in which a black perspective is vital to the care of black children. Many white-led homes focus on attachment and separation work with children in a way that negates the value of relationships they may have. It is commonly assumed that a child cannot be 'attached' to a parent or grandparent who lives a long way away and whom the child has not seen for a long time. However, black staff had a different understanding based on the knowledge that because of immigration controls, colonisation etc, black people have developed the capacity to maintain relationships over vast distances in time and miles, and consequently worked with the child in maintaining the relationships that were important to the child. Similarly in placing children in alternative families, white workers have often based their practice on the belief that a child won't settle or become attached unless they have been psychologically 'separated' from former carers. A black perspective on this issue as highlighted by the study is one that promotes the concept of shared care and that attachments need not be mutually exclusive. It is interesting that this concept has now been taken on and is a fundamental aspect of the Children Act 1989. The key worker system is also valuable since it provides residents with a sense of continuity. However, this should not occur in isolation from interaction with other staff, as the effects of staff sickness and annual leave have to be taken account of, and planned for accordingly.

Whatever system is used within the home, it is vital that the care provided ensures that each resident has an appropriate worker with particular responsibility for meeting their needs.

The reliance of the projects on a community approach embodies the principles and practice of multi-disciplinary working and flexible, participative management styles.

It is an approach that was demonstrated by:

—the utilisation of youth workers for outside activities;

—teachers and social workers as night staff; and

—outside workers to establish carers' support groups.

The involvement of teachers in projects is based on the belief that education is crucial to the survival of black people. Local authority schools have a history of rejecting black young people through labelling them and dismissing their potential in various ways. Teachers in some projects have been involved in additional teaching, to facilitate the re-entry of children into mainstream schools. Our experience generally of children in care is that workers have low expectations of them educationally. Black workers were not willing to accept this view of the children in their care, believing that it contributes to low self-esteem and as such cannot be a feature of genuine care.

The relationship of staff with residents was perceived as fundamentally different to that which is experienced within a local authority setting. One way in which this was reflected was in the roles which workers undertake having a 'fluidity' as opposed to the 'rigidity' often experienced. Flexible use of staff enhanced the services available to residents, and also enabled the staff to further the development of their skills. The ethos of the staff/residents relationship was based on respect for the person, not their job or job title. This approach leads to a less hierarchical atmosphere, which was preferred by residents and staff. The resident/staff relationship also mirrors the experience of the community, for example there is a respect for elders. Elders in the residential establishments regarded the staff 'like their children', but also recognised the boundaries of the relationship. Similarly, staff in children's homes have a sense of parental responsibility for the young people in their care. The belief of staff that 'yes, I do expect a lot from you', as opposed to having low or no expectations, led to a situation in which young people were able to develop their potential. The parental role of staff was over and above the usual more limited role of residential social workers. One of the features of black-led homes is that unlike their white counterparts, black workers are more likely to live within the community of the home. As a consequence, their relationship with the young people extends beyond the walls of the homes. It was quite usual, in fact expected and valued, that workers off duty and seeing young people out on the streets would still be 'caring' for them, reprimanding them for misbehavour etc. Black staff often expressed the view that to allow young people too much freedom under the auspices of 'trust' and 'independence' was a liberal approach they could not afford. As black adults they were aware of the criminalisation of black young people, plus the dangers of drugs, harassment etc, and had a responsibility to support and protect them out of the home. This approach was expected and welcomed by young people's families. Elders did not view themselves as passive recipients of care, but as having an active role in the development of services to them, and ensuring a good quality of life for each other, as well as the workers and their families.

4. MANAGEMENT

The management structure of the projects visited varied. In some projects, management were part of the staff group, whilst in others, the management committee facilitated the management function. In some of the projects, people fulfilled both roles, where staff were also part of the management committee. The need for a community approach is reflected in project management committees, through which individuals provide a link for the projects to the community.

Management committees, while often providing a source of support, can also be a source of conflict and stress. There was evidence of this within some of the projects in the study. Conflict can lead to debate and development, and when constructively handled can have positive spin-offs for the management committee and the project. However, it may also adversely affect the operation of the committee and will have an influence on decisions taken by this body. And taken in conjunction with other factors such as under-resourcing, the affects of management committee conflict can be exacerbated.

Some of the management committees involved in the study maintained a flexible approach. They provided the structures for financial and managerial accountability, a forum to debate ideas and produce plans, a means through which problems could be solved and a system for linking the work of the projects to other community initiatives. The members of committees were often actively involved in the projects and visited regularly to talk to staff and residents.

The under-funding of black projects has a direct effect on managers. Many of them have to spend a disproportionate amount of time in seeking funding and lobbying to maintain it. Their responsibilities are greatly increased as a consequence and other tensions develop as they are not able to allocate enough time to other management functions. The creativity and flexibility of black projects was much in evidence through the management systems also. Their imaginative approach was evident in obtaining and utilising resources. It is ironic then that the local authorities use the excuse that there are not enough black people with management experience to justify their unwillingness to employ black managers. The scenario is indicative of the statutory sector attitude in under-valuing the experience of management in any other sectors, and also of the undervaluing of the work of black projects generally.

5. FINANCE

That black projects are under-funded cannot be disputed. However there are other issues which affect the financial position of projects. In sharing some of their experiences, the black projects highlighted some of these issues.

The study revealed that the majority of projects were not being adequately recompensed for the services they were providing. This leads to a situation where there is a need for services on the one hand, and projects willing to provide them on the other, but the finance is not made available to ensure that this happens. Inevitably, it is the potential or actual user of services who is affected most by this process.

Another aspect of finance is that funding bodies often apply conditions which conflict with the aims of the project. This is illustrated by the client-based approach of funders, ie provision for funding for projects for elders, children etc, rather than the community-based, holistic approach advocated by black projects. A further example is the condition that projects must seek alternative sources of funding. This not only leads to frustration, as so little funding is forthcoming, but also means that time spent on seeking funding distracts members of the organisation from other more creative work they could undertake.

Black projects have a history and continuing reality of uncertainty surrounding their funding situation. They are often on short term or minimal funding, which hampers potential developments. Funding bodies seem prone to shortsightedness especially in relation to black projects and this, coupled with a lack of awareness of the changing needs of black communities, has led to many projects having to take in a greater amount of work than their resources can support or else being unable to meet needs. While the projects are constantly reviewing the needs of the residents because of their close community needs, funders do not generally review (except to determine whether to continue funding) the funding needs of the project.

Local authorities pay a pittance for good quality care provided by black organisations. This contrasts sharply with white 'specialist' homes which receive much higher fees for the services which they provide. Clearly, this illustrates an undervaluing of services provided by black projects. The experience black people have of the welfare system directly impacts upon the financial resources of black organisations. Many black elders do not receive the benefits of full pensions or because of immigration rules etc cannot claim severe disablement allowances. Black-led homes frequently find that they are unable to charge the full rates to residents because of this. A positive dimension of the black perspective in residential care is that black staff are often well aware of the financial situation of black elders and take it into account, even if it means that the project's own finances are depleted as a result. We are left wondering whether the charging policies of local authorities, with the implementation of the NHS and Community Care Act, will also take into account the financial position of black people. The picture was a similar one with regard to young people again based on the knowledge that black young people are both more likely to be unemployed and even when they are employed, more likely to receive lower wages than white people of the same age, and therefore projects were unlikely to recover full charges for care provided.

6. LOCATION

The location of the home is important not only for the residents, but also for their families. The choice of location, when part of the black community, enables residents to feel safe and comfortable both within and outside the home. Within other communities, black people are more likely to experience racial harassment and abuse. Location of the home was seen as crucial in helping young black people to maintain their identity and give them a sense of belonging.

The experience of those projects catering for black young men was that white people in the surrounding community had stereotyped images of the black male as being involved with drugs, crime etc. These views were then manifested through continual complaints to the police, who in collusion maintained a high profile in the vicinity of the home on a regular basis, thereby reinforcing the stereotype.

The study highlighted a common experience shared by the black projects which was that there was resistance from all white communities to the establishment of black homes in the area. However, professional classes were able to use systems they had knowledge of to hinder or stop developments, for example the use of professional and local political networks. Projects pointed out that the development of a relationship between the home and the local community is critical. This should be part of a continuum, occurring both before the home is set up, and once the project is established. It was important to organise meetings and attend meetings as well as to arrange social events that brought people from the community and the home together. This was a means of maintaining a positive relationship and keeping the community informed of the progress of the project.

Section Two

A Focus of Good Practice?

In sharing their experiences and knowledge, the eight projects highlighted a broad spectrum of issues which have clear implications for local authorities, funding bodies and residential establishments alike. The most fundamental of the issues highlighted is the philosophy which underpins the work of black-led organisations. A philosophy developed from black histories, cultural experiences and resistance to racism/oppression. A philosophy based on a view of life and the world which acknowledges the wholeness of the being and does not compartmentalise their behaviour, experiences, needs, expectations, cultures into neat and separate boxes.

We believe there is much to learn from the experiences of black organisations and we hope local authorities and other organisations will begin to value the experiences and expertise of these organisations. The starting point must surely be in white organisations examining the ethos and culture of their own organisation. Do they provide services and practice that devalue black people and consistently fail to see them, their experiences, and their cultures in any contextual framework? Perhaps this will result in a more critical analysis of the way in which white individuals and institutions operate with black individuals and organisations. We believe that development of positive partnerships with black voluntary organisations, a part of legislative requirements, would be one way of developing models of good practice based on the experience of black projects.

If local authorities and other organisations are to provide a more equitable service to all the communities, then services to black communities must of necessity be high on their agenda. To this end, agencies should support and encourage the development of more black-led residential establishments, and begin to incorporate some of the philosophies and models identified by black professionals, communities and organisations, into the establishment of 'good practice'.

Recommendations

Residential homes should:

1. Have clear aims and objectives, outlining who they are providing a service to and what that service is; the service must reflect the needs of black residents.

2. Have a black perspective fully integrated into all policies and practices.

3. Ensure that the recruitment of staff reflects the community reality and the needs of the residents.

4. Ensure that the staff have an understanding of the realities and needs of black residents.

5. Develop links with and support black organisations and individuals within the community.

6. Develop processes of supervision of staff which incorporate exploration of race and cultural dimensions.

7. Meet all the physical needs of the residents; this includes health, skin care, food and language.

8. Ensure that they are able to communicate with residents and their families in a means and language which they feel comfortable with.

9. Ensure that care builds on the positive strengths of black people.

10. Respect residents' practices of faith, and make the necessary arrangements for them to fulfil these.

11. Develop relationships with the local community which will enrich the lives of residents.

Local authorities and funding bodies MUST:

12. Ensure that assessment procedures and processes incorporate the black reality.

13. Make available to residents and potential residents information necessary to enable them to make personal choices.

14. Establish and maintain fruitful partnership relationships with black projects.

15. Ensure that black projects are supported, not only in terms of financial concerns, but also other broader resource issues, eg training.

16. Review their terms and conditions of funding to guard against the abuse of black projects.

Brief Bibliography

Ahmad, A., *Social Services for Black People: Service or Lip Service?* Rev, 1988

Hughes, R. D., *Social Services for Ethnic Minorities: Policy and Practice in the North West*, DHSS/SSI, 1986

Jones, A., *Report of the Black Communities Care Project*, NISW, 1991

Jones, A., Phillips, M., Maynard, C., *A Home From Home*, NISW, 1992

Black Perspectives Sub-Group:

Adele Jones
National Institute for Social Work

Charles Maynard
Bradford Social Services

Marcia Richards
Race Equality Unit

Daphne Statham
Chairman

CHAPTER SEVEN

Staffing Arrangements in Residential Care

Sub-Group Report

Introduction

The Staffing Arrangements Sub-Group was commissioned to draw up a handbook of guidance for managers, proprietors, employers and trade union officers involved in residential care, in order to implement the final recommendation of the Wagner Report: 'The DHSS should identify ways in which residential staffing requirements may best be calculated and how staff may best be deployed.' The handbook 'Staffing in Residential Care Homes', was published by NISW in 1990, and has been widely used in all types of settings. The text presented here is based on the handbook, but also incorporates comment and feedback received from readers.

The organisation of staffing certainly has to take some account of staff needs, but its prime purpose has to be the meeting of residents' needs. This can be seen in many ways. If residents feel constrained to go to bed early or to get up early, in order to make life a little easier for hardpressed staff, they do not have a real choice about bedtimes or getting-up times, regardless of what published regulations say. If residents are not allowed to dress themselves because it takes too long, this too infringes their control over their own lives. If time cannot be made available for residents with learning disabilities to have individualised social skills training, their potential to manage for themselves may never be realised. If there is no staff member free to talk out a problem with a child at the time the child needs to talk, it will be an opportunity lost to resolve problems and make progress. In all these cases, the quality of service that can be offered, and the choices available to residents, are affected by the number of staff, and how they are deployed.

Residential care homes vary enormously. Some of the differences are obvious, such as the size or the characteristics of the group of people who live in the home. Others are less obvious, but anyone who has visited homes will know that even two homes which are apparently identical in design and staffing will have different characteristics. The aim of the Sub-Group in preparing the handbook was not to reduce or ignore that variety but, in giving general guidance on staffing arrangements, to recognise the different aims and natures of homes, and provide a framework as widely applicable as possible, in principle aimed at homes of all sizes, for all client groups, and for people of every level of dependence and independence.

The handbook was also intended to be practical. There is no single right answer to many staffing problems. Often it is necessary to compromise, for example in balancing cost against the desired levels of staffing cover. However, it has to be recognised that staff are the prime resource of any residential home. Staffing levels must ensure that residents have a way of life which is not dominated by limitations concerning staffing, such as rotas, and that staff are not exploited, and have sufficient support to minimise the incidence of violence and stress. These are issues which employers and managers must take seriously, primarily for the sake of the residents, but also out of concern for staff and in order to comply with legislation such as the Health and Safety at Work Act. If issues concerning staffing are discussed fully at an early stage, they may be resolved to the mutual advantage of managers, staff and residents before they can become problems.

What the handbook tried to do was to offer a level-headed way of tackling these problems; facing the issues may not produce perfect solutions, but a recognition of the problems involved should lead to greater understanding and, perhaps, alternative ways of dealing with them. The intention was to achieve a balance between sensitivity to the complex needs of residents and the presentation of an approach reasonably simple, comprehensible and easy to apply.

In the sections following, the stages of setting up a home in terms of its staffing establishment are considered, identifying the basic principles involved and spelling out the practical considerations of applying the principles. The original handbook also lists questions which need to be borne in mind by way of checklists, and finally gives some worked examples, as illustrations for readers of how the methods proposed might be used to make calculations or staffing proposals in their own settings.

In the feedback received since the handbook was first published, there has been a request for minimum standards to be identified. Clearly there are strong arguments for setting minimum standards, if only to assist in the processes of registration and inspection. There are also fears that the minimum might become the norm. Furthermore, the variety of homes means their such calculations could become extremely complex. This area remains one which will warrant further research and debate.

The conventional 'staffing ratios' (x Residents: y Staff) approach was avoided by the Sub-Group as too rigid. Instead, a way of thinking about staffing arrangements was devised to help those involved in the planning was to help become aware of the issues, and discuss them objectively. It is of vital importance to staff and residents alike to get the estabishment and deployment of staff right. If there are too few staff, they will be overworked and risk providing poor standards of care; if too many, so that they are underworked, there are, in fact, similar risks. Many potential problems can be avoided by consultation. Prospective proprietors need to involve registration officers at an early stage as the staffing costs will have a major effect on their budgets. Employers and managers need to consult trades unions and staff representatives to ensure that the welfare of the workforce and the practitioners' views are considered.

In the end, though, the staff are there to serve the residents, and the outcome of the calculations and consultations has to be to ensure that residents' needs are met in the most appropriate way.

Section One

The Home and the Residents

1. WHAT IS THE HOME FOR?

The aims and objectives of each residential care home must be clearly laid down. Aims are long term, overall targets which may not necessarily be attained but show the general intentions and give a sense of direction; objectives, by contrast, are specific and achievable.

It may be helpful first to spell out the general philosophy, values and even belief system that underlie the aims of the establishment. Examples of general aims are 'helping people compensate for disability', 'enabling people to become more independent', or 'assisting children to develop and cope with their social and emotional problems'. Examples of specific objectives are 'offering personal care in feeding, dressing and hygiene', 'providing programmes of independence training', or 'running group counselling sessions'. The working methods of the establishment should be based upon the philosophy, aims and objectives, and should also be made explicit.

It is a requirement of registration that homes must have a statement of their aims, and these should be laid down in a brochure for residents and their families. The staffing of a home obviously needs to be geared up to fulfil its aims, and the aims therefore need to be written up in a way which leads logically to the staffing needed. The most acute level of service to be offered needs to be spelt out so that staffing can be geared to match. Even the smallest homes where residents need to be lifted require at least two staff actively on duty at all times, for example.

Levels of need with which the staff will not normally have to deal need to be spelt out. It should also be known to all staff what support is available in the event of crises or unusual demands upon them beyond those that may normally be expected. Homes where confused residents may wander and put themselves at risk will need sufficient staff to accompany or monitor them, if other devices such as tagging or locked doors are to be avoided. Where people may be unpredictably violent, staffing levels need to suffice to give reasonable protection to both staff and residents. Homes where residents are being encouraged to be independent and do things for themselves may need similar levels of staffing to those for more dependent people, as it may take longer to teach, encourage and observe residents do something for themselves than to do it for them.

It should be made clear to potential residents and their families prior to admission what their rights and responsibilities are. It should be made quite explicit what kind of care the home is able to provide, which needs it cannot meet, and what arrangements will be made if a resident's needs become more than the home can cope with. The aim should be to maintain residents in the home as long as possible, and in the event of greater levels of dependence, it is preferable if additional support can be obtained rather than discharge a resident. However, if a home cannot continue to provide for a resident, the reasons should be made clear and adequate notice given both to the resident and to their immediate family.

The clarification of aims and objectives needs particular emphasis when setting up a new residential care home. If done badly, the rest of the process will fall apart. Similarly, where homes change their functions over a period without explicitly changing their aims and objectives, it is quite possible for the staffing to be inadequate for the task, but if the home's aims and objectives were not made clear originally, changes cannot be identified so easily, and the consequences in terms of changed staffing needs are not so obvious.

In some homes for older people, staffing levels still relate to a time when residents were generally fitter and more lucid; greater clarity about the target group of residents would reveal the creeping change towards increased confusion and frailty, and the need to adapt staffing arrangements. There are still children's homes staffed to meet the needs of young children with limited presenting problems while the homes now deal with teenagers with complex difficulties: the change may well have taken place over a period of years.

Some changes may be temporary: a person with terminal illness may need a level of care beyond the normal staffing establishment, which can be augmented temporarily to match the increased need. Some homes have cyclical demands, such as children's homes where a large proportion of the residents go home at weekends. Some hostels for people with learning disabilities may face extra pressure during ATC holiday weeks. Again, the demand for respite care of all types tends to peak at holiday periods.

Homes sometimes have more than one role, and there can be inconsistencies or tensions between them. It is important to make them explicit. In addition to providing care for its residents, a home may offer day care, or other services; its premises may be used to provide meals on wheels, or house a team of staff unconnected with the home. The home may take students on practical placements regularly; it may be the home of resident staff. All these secondary functions may have implications for staffing, as well as for other aspects of the home's life.

The home's working methods also need to be made clear, since they will indicate what type of staff are required to fulfil the home's functions. The working style of homes varies considerably. In some, duties are shared widely, with assistant staff acting as keyworkers for example, while in others senior staff bear all the responsibilities. Account may need to be taken of services made available locally, for example by the health service or local authority. If not available on a normal basis, special arrangements may need to be made. These services include home tuition, chiropody, occupational therapy and community nursing.

2. WHAT SORT OF PERSON WILL LIVE IN THE HOME?

Staff need to have the range of skills, knowledge and experience required to match the range of residents' needs. Most residents live in homes grouped with other residents with similar needs because it is easier to provide for them when grouped together in this way. The problems they share in common tend to become the dominant feature, and staff skills, knowledge and experience will need to be matched to compensate for, or alleviate, their needs.

Older people form the largest client group in residential care, and staff in such homes are expected to deal with the range of infirmities from which older people may suffer. (Being old is not a disability in itself). Some homes may be for people with specific disabilities such as people with deafness and blindness. Other homes may be process-orientated, whether for one client group or more, such as assessment centres for children, respite care units for people with mental handicaps, pre-independence units or holiday homes. Many homes serve more than one client group or fulfil different functions in different units. Homes may contain people from ethnic, cultural or religious groups which will require special consideration in staffing arrangements.

Whether homes have broad or specialist functions, the staff team will need to have a wide variety of skills which all need to be identified. The full range of skill areas needs to be listed, including management, administration, nursing education, personal care, counselling, groupwork, rehabilitation and skills training and leisure activities. For homes which are already running, the staff team may need to be modified from time to time to match the residents' changing needs. In some cases this will reflect growing dependence or independence as people get older. In other cases, the initial assessment of a new resident prior to admission may indicate the need for additional skills not already available.

Some of the skills may be needed all the time, some at regular intervals and some occasionally. The main needs of the primary client group will indicate the basic mode of the home and the nature of the core staff. For example intensive personal care for older people will require the core staffing to be care workers, whereas in therapeutic units for people recovering from mental illness, there may be a need for residential social workers specially trained in the home's systems. While the core staff are likely to be needed at all times to provide basic care or supervision, other staff will be needed at intervals, such as administrative staff in office hours only, or consultant psychiatrists visiting on demand.

When people live in their own homes, their needs may be met by members of their family or neighbours, by volunteers or paid staff, and there is often an overlap between these groups. If people move into residential care, this balance will shift towards paid staff, but consideration still needs to be given to the provision of community services of the type normally enjoyed by people in their own homes, either within the home or through access to services in the community.

Residents' initial care plans on entering homes should indicate the range of services they need, and admission should not be grounds for penalising them through the withdrawal of services available to them in their own homes. It is possible for homes to be attended by a medical practitioner who visits regularly; alternatively each resident may choose to have his or her own doctor. Consideration needs to be given to the home's policy on the recruitment and deployment of volunteers.

Depending upon the management style and working methods of the home, services can be provided in various ways. For example, all staff may think they do counselling, whereas only a small number of staff may be trained to counsel. It needs to be made explicit whether the home is reliant on staff to respond intuitively to problems, or whether specific keyworkers are identified and trained to deal with residents' personal problems, or whether in-depth counselling is left to specialist visiting experts, such as psychologists or psychiatrists.

3. HOW MANY PEOPLE IS THE HOME FOR?

Staff need to have the right skills, knowledge and experience in the right volume to match the scale of residents' needs. Residents should live in groups of no more than 16 persons in size, and, indeed, smaller groups are preferable if institutional living is to be avoided. Some homes have, in any case, fewer than 16 residents, and will need to be considered as one group, unless they happen to be subdivided into smaller units. Homes that serve more than 16 residents will need to be divided internally to provide smaller groupings, such as a home for 40 elderly people being subdivided into four groups of 10.

Groups or units may have different purposes. In some homes, units may be used for specific functions, such as admission or rehabilitation. In others they may serve different groups of residents, with a unit set aside for severely confused older people, or for people with multiple handicaps needing extra care. The more specialist the unit, the more expert the staff can become, but such units can also be very artificial and abnormal. There are arguments both for and against the integration and segregation of residents with special needs.

One of the main purposes of dividing homes into units is to ensure that residents have access to the care most appropriate to their individual needs. Ensuring vital continuity of care by a small team of staff is facilitated by such units. For each unit or group, the number of core staff required at any one time needs to be identified, taking account of the range of problems that can reasonably be anticipated in the normal running of the home. A chart can be produced for each unit to show peaks and troughs in demand.

There is no absolutely correct staffing for each unit, but various factors need to be borne in mind in coming to a decision. The amount of physical work to be done, the need for individual attention, peaks in demand, the likelihood of control problems, additional duties such as the escorting of individuals outside the home all need to be considered. It is also essential to maintain a degree of flexibility to cover the unforeseen difficulties which inevitably crop up in residential work, and which make the job so demanding and fascinating.

Any mechanistic approach to the subject is likely to fail; calculating the length of time it takes a care assistant to bath a resident, for example, can put at risk the value of using the occasion as a leisurely and relaxed opportunity for the resident to chat privately. Peaks and troughs in demand should be based on the needs and wishes of residents rather than staff. Breakfasts should be timed to suit elderly residents, for example; this may entail flexible mealtimes with people coming and going as they choose, rather than a restricted approach with fixed times.

Within the spectrum of provision, there are very wide variations. At one end are the units for people presenting the greatest demands, such as secure units for children, where a high level of staffing has to be maintained at all times. At the other are cluster units for people with learning disabilities and homes akin to sheltered accommodation for older people, where the staffing input may be limited to occasional visits or the provision of a warden or housekeeper.

In some homes, more than one chart may need to be completed, for example when there are different patterns of demand for staffing at different times of the week or year (eg term-time as against weekends or school holidays in a children's home). In such cases, calculation will have to be made pro rata for the different patterns of work. It is at this stage that consultation with staff and trades unions is most critical if work loads are to make sense on the ground.

The day staffing needs of a home should allow for days off, holidays, staff meetings, handover, staff training and some sick leave; a home staffed in this way should not need external staffing support except in extreme crisis, such as a flu epidemic or multiple vacancies. As for night staffing, this is often reduced to the minimum consistent with maintaining the oversight of the home. Where residents are lucid, fit and do not present major behavioural problems, sleeping-in staff may suffice. Back-up systems should, however, be identified in case of crisis, expecially where staffing is reduced at nights, or where people left in charge have limited experience, training or authority.

Where residents may need help, cover needs to cope with demands that can be anticipated in the normal running of the home, such as lifting (where two staff are needed), illness, wandering, enuresis, nightmares, night-time admissions and deaths. It is not always possible to provide sufficient staff to cope with total fire evacuation; the brigade and other sources of help need to be contacted, and staffing levels have to be sufficient to ensure that contact can be made.

Consideration also has to be given, depending on the circumstances, to the security of the building, staff and residents, to maintenance duties, and to work that may be undertaken by staff at night, such as some domestic duties.

Sleeping-in duties are not popular now in local authority work, but are much more common in the private sector. If senior managers are present at night, it is possible to monitor night staff more closely, and ensure consistency of practice with day shifts. However, sleeping in on call can be unsettling and tiring, and if staff are resident at the home, they may find that too many demands are made on them and that it is difficult to get time off. There are also still a few homes where staff and their families are resident in order to create a family atmosphere; where this happens, care will need to be taken to ensure that the secondary purpose of creating a home for the staff does not detract from the primary purpose of creating a home for the residents.

In some cases, a smaller team of highly experienced or trained staff may be more effective than a larger inexperienced or untrained staff. This is particularly true where relationships with residents require skilled handling, for example in dealing with disturbed adolescents.

Allowance needs to be made if the home fulfils functions not related to the residents, or if staff have other duties, so that the time available for residents is not diminished. If the home is used as a training base for staff, allowance will need to be made for training sessions and student supervision.

Individual staff members who are magistrates, councillors, trade union officials or officers of professional bodies may need additional time off regularly. Some staff may need maternity leave, or substantial compassionate leave. Similarly, students on secondment for training may be away all or part of the time, depending upon the format of the course. Unless these absences are limited or very occasional, the staff team will need to be augmented to compensate or standards of care will fall below the level acknowledged as being necessary.

Staffing may need to be reassessed from time to time. The level of independence and dependence of residents may vary, and staffing may need to be increased or decreased depending upon circumstances. For example, a children's home where it is assumed that all children will be at school will be inadequately staffed to provide all-day cover for unemployed older children. People with learning disabilities may need less support as they achieve greater independence and develop improved social skills. Again, the residents of a home for the elderly may become imperceptibly more frail and confused.

Section Two

Staff Support and Organisation

1. HOW SHOULD THE STAFF BE SUPPORTED?

Staff need the training and support systems to ensure they have the right skills, knowledge and experience. Residential work can be both demanding and stressful. To meet its demands and cope with the stress, staff need to be adequately provided with support. Some of the support will be provided by colleagues in the home, or by line managers. However, consideration needs to be given to other sources of help.

Staff may need individual supervision and/or group supervision, depending upon the nature of the home. Where a keyworker system is in operation, and individual staff carry specific responsibilities in relation to individual residents, their work as keyworkers will require supervision to ensure accountability and offer support. Some homes have consultant advisers to provide guidance and support; for example, social workers in the local authority, family practitioners and other health service staff, or external advisers and consultants. Such advisers may need to be seen as a part of the staff team. Registration officers may also offer advice.

If the home is already in operation, attention should be given to staff wastage, and to sickness rates, as these may be indicators that staff support systems or additional training are required. Exit interviews with staff leaving can help to identify stress if they feel able to speak freely. Recruitment difficulties can also be a pointer towards the image of a home, or of the agency, as a supportive employer. Trades unions and professional associations can offer support to their members in residential homes, and their officers may need time off to fulfil their duties in helping to resolve problems.

Staff in residential homes require adequate training both before they enter the work, and on an in-service basis. Some staff need to be trained to qualification level. The pattern of training currently being developed under the National Council for Vocational Qualifications recognises a number of levels of skill to match levels of responsibility and complexity of task. However, the picture is not yet clear, and it would be inappropriate to be prescriptive about the training levels and types required.

It may be necessary in some homes to ensure that a qualified person is on duty at all times, in order to ensure that there is the appropriate cover for emergencies or complex situations. In others a qualified person may be needed to provide frequent supervision without needing to be available at all times.

Depending upon the nature of the establishment, each home should have a training plan, which should include: initial induction training matched to each post; consolidatory training to reinforce induction; ongoing in-service training opportunities for individual

staff; team training exercises; and opportunities to undertake qualifying courses.

Initial induction training needs to include statutory requirements such as health and safety training, and the information and
skills needed for staff to cope with a new job. When new working
methods or new developments are introduced, they should be
preceded by appropriate training, so that staff always feel confident
that they know what to do and how to do it.

As with consultant advice, training may be provided by a variety
of people, including both external and internal trainers. Training
takes many forms, including seminars, group teaching, placements,
reading and so on; residential work provides excellent opportunities for teacher and student to work together and share learning. Training must take account of the needs of ethnic, cultural and
religious groups.

Training takes time and is therefore expensive. However, it
should be seen as a necessary cost and built into the budget. An
average of five working days per annum per member of staff is not
unreasonable, although the actual amount will depend upon the
complexity of jobs and the needs of individual staff.

2. HOW SHOULD STAFF BE ORGANISED?

The organisation of staff has to take account primarily of residents'
needs, but also of the needs of staff. In devising rotas for staff, it is
necessary to start from the needs of the residents, and to attempt to
meet them wherever possible. Account also has to be taken, however, of staff needs if they are to be recruited and retained. If shifts
start or finish too late or too early, transport to work may be difficult
or expensive, and travelling may be (or feel) dangerous and off-
putting for staff.

Staff should have clear information concerning management's
expectations about the hours they are to work in writing at the time
of their appointment, even if changes in the task of the home may
require subsequent changes. Some homes do live from hand to
mouth, with rotas being devised day by day. It is important,
however, to plan well in advance, with a skeleton rota which can be
modified if necessary: planning saves time and resources, and staff
know where they stand.

Some staff prefer a rotating rota, with varying shifts. Others
prefer to work mornings, or evenings, or weekends. Some flexibility
can be built in to meet staff needs, as long as the primary purpose of

the home is recognised, and the dog wags the tail. Where changes are planned, staff should be consulted. If staff have an understanding of the thinking behind the rota, then there is much better chance of co-operation, expecially when their goodwill is needed at crisis times. Regular times off permit staff to plan their private lives, which makes demands on their families more acceptable.

Careful planning is also needed in relation to holiday times. In children's homes, school holidays can create peak demand, coinciding with the periods when staff may wish to take their leave. If residents are not to suffer, the maintenance of basic staffing at such times is vital. Temporary arrangements can help, such as the appointment of extra staff during the summer months, or increasing the hours of part-timers to cover absences or increased demand. Split shifts put additional pressure on staff and are not now generally acceptable; computers can be useful in devising skeleton rotas.

Rotas need to take realistic account of the demands of the work. There needs to be a built-in handover period in order for staff to share information and ensure continuity of care without having to rely on staff goodwill to provide the time needed. It can be helpful to establish a regular co-ordinating day when as many staff as possible are available for staff meetings, staff training, supervision and planning.

Rotas need to take account of agreed conditions of service, such as the current 39-hour week in local authority homes, and the five day working week. These have been negotiated to make the work manageable; excessive hours risk leaving staff exhausted and in danger of acting inappropriately, causing harm to residents, because of undue stress.

Rotas also need to provide reasonable conditions that have not been formally covered in negotiations. For example, it is generally accepted that staff should have regular weekends off, with one in three as the minimum. Split shifts are no longer acceptable in most homes, although there are some circumstances, such as in residential schools, where they may be specially negotiated as part of a specific package of conditions. Arrangements have to be made for cover during breaks in shifts and staff meal times, including breaks for night staff.

Staffing arrangements must be checked against the perceptions of the residents. It is the job of proprietors and senior managers to arrange back-up staffing. A system may be very efficient as far as staff are concerned, but make life unhappy from the residents' viewpoint. For example, rotas may require residents to get up or go to bed too early, or lead to impersonal institutional patterns of bathing, dressing or toiletting. When a rota is being proposed, its consequences for individual residents need to be considered before it is adopted. If staff due to take over at handover time are not available, perhaps through sudden illness, it is not the responsibility of assistant staff to find replacements before they go off duty, but to alert those to whom they are accountable.

The balance of part-time and full-time staff needs to be considered carefully, as an imbalance can affect the quality of care. The appointment of too many full-timers can lead to less flexibility of rotas, for example in seeking replacement staff in the event of sudden illness. A predominance of part-time staff can lead to complications in the sheer number of staff. Each part-timer needs as much training as a full-timer, and staff meetings use up a greater percentage of their time. If too many staff relate to a resident, it can diminish their dignity and individuality through the sharing of intimate functions and personal matters too widely. Lack of full-time posts can also lose experienced part-timers who wish to move to full-time work.

Consideration needs to be given to the balance of responsibilities in a staff team. In a small home the officer in charge or manager has to be a jack-of-all-trades. In larger homes, however, it is possible to specialise, with senior staff acting as domestic bursar or head of care, for example, and with specialist ancillary roles such as laundry worker. Again, it may help to amalgamate the roles of care assistants and domestics if small staff teams are to provide integrated care for smaller groups in homes for the elderly.

This chapter has laid out the issues which have to be considered in creating a staff team to match the tasks it has to carry out. The detailed formulae and draft forms for making calculations were included in the handbook prepared by the Wagner Development Group and published by the National Institute for Social Work. Clearly it is a subject on which there is no single simple right answer, but it is also a subject of real importance if residents' needs are to be met.

Brief Bibliography

Barr, H., *Perspectives on Training For Residential Work*, CCETSW, 1987

Care-Sector Consortium, *Residential Domiciliary and Day Care Project*, Care Sector Consortium, 1989

Social Care Association, *Staffing Ratios*, SCA 1980

Wagner Development Group, *Staffing in Residential Care Homes*, NISW, 1990.

Wagner Development Group
Staffing Arrangements Sub-Group

Harry Barker
National Union of Public Employees

Stephen Campbell
Association of County Councils

Richard Clough
Chairman, Social Care Association

Christina Craig
National Council for Voluntary Organisations

Ross Greig
British Federation of Care Home Proprietors

Brian Jones
Association of Metropolitan Authorities

Des Kelly
Social Care Association

David Lane
Association of Directors of Social Service

Sheila McGrath
British Association of Social Workers

Alison Mitchell
National Association of Local Government Officers

Christine Peaker
   National Council for Voluntary Organisations (November
      1988–March 1989)

Sheila Scott
   National Care Homes Association

Jane Woodwark
   Local Authorities Conditions of Service Advisory Board

CHAPTER 8

The Caring in Homes Initiative

Penny Youll, Brunel University

The Caring in Homes Initiative (CHI) makes a number of important contributions to the 'positive answers' that have flowed from the Wagner Review.[1] The Initiative was set up in February 1989 by the Department of Health as a three year programme of developmental research which aimed to demonstrate how several of the recommendations and issues highlighted by the Wagner Review might be put into practice.

Over 250 care homes, involving all client groups, were involved in practical projects across the country. These included homes run by private companies, owner proprietors, small local voluntary organisations, large national voluntary agencies and homes run by local authorities. The results of CHI do, therefore, draw on a very wide range and diversity of experience and interests: it is this which helps to give the outcomes of the research authority and relevance.

Four agencies were commissioned to develop ways of promoting good residential care and management practice with the aim of helping to ensure a high quality of life for residents. The four programmes of research focused on: training for care staff, the links between care homes and their local community, in-house review and self-evaluation, and the provision of information for service users. This chapter gives an account of each of those programmes in turn and highlights some of the lessons which can be drawn from CHI as a whole.

The author heads the group at Brunel University which has conducted an independent evaluation of the Initiative for the Department of Health: a full account of this work will be published later in 1993.[2]

General Features

Before discussing each of the main Programmes, it is helpful to set out one or two of the key features of the Caring in Homes Initiative.

First of all, the aim of the research was to find ways of improving quality of life by promoting good practice. This was done not only by taking account of existing guidelines and recommendations; the researchers also put emphasis on the contribution that residents and their relatives could make in clarifying the purposes of care homes, shaping the way homes are run and helping to set and review standards.

A second feature of CHI was that the work was conducted in close collaboration with front-line workers in care establishments and, wherever possible, residents themselves. The aim was to ensure that the materials produced would be relevant and practical since they would be shaped very directly by the experience of service providers.

Like the Wagner Review, the work of CHI was concerned with all the main care groups: care homes for elderly people, for people with learning difficulties, for people with mental health problems, for people with physical disabilities and sensory impairment, for people with drug or alcohol problems and homes for children and young people. The aim was that the approaches explored by the research would, as far as possible, be adaptable and useful across the care groups.

1. INSIDE QUALITY ASSURANCE

Internal Review and Self Evaluation

One of the key recommendations of the Wagner Review concerned the importance of independent inspection and review.

Although the Review strongly advocated that all establishments should be subject to the same system of registration and inspection the review did not consider that this would be sufficient to set and maintain high standards: periodic internal review was also required.

The Wagner Review was clear that providers '. . . should promote systems of self-evaluation and performance review . . . no new establishment should be registered which is not prepared to adopt such a system,', and that these should include, as well as staff at all levels, 'the expressed wishes and views of residents and their relatives.'[3]

The message was, therefore, that formal inspections and external reviews, while essential, were unlikely to deliver and maintain appropriate standards: it was necessary to establish responsibility for ongoing review of aims and performance within the care home and to involve residents and their relatives in the process.

The Centre for Environmental and Social Studies of Ageing (CESSA) at the Polytechnic of North London (now the University of North London) was commissioned to develop a system of internal review which would meet these requirements and which could be used independently by agencies and care home managers. The programme adopted the title 'Inside Quality Assurance' (IQA) to emphasise the point that the system to be developed was about carrying out an in-house review. The responsibility for initiating the process and deciding how to respond to the results would lie, in the first instance, within the care home.

The CESSA programme was strongly committed to the values of residents' rights and the promotion of residents' wellbeing. They had established a rationale for taking residents' needs, views and ideas as the key both to the work of development and to the implementation of the system itself.[4] The comments and views of residents were taken as the most important but not the only source of information for a review of quality.

The Challenge

There were several challenges to be faced in developing any system of internal review but especially one which would involve residents and care workers at all levels.

First, the studies of the CESSA team[5] show how reticent direct service users are in commenting on their experience. The reasons for this are well-known: people do not want to risk upsetting those on whom they depend for their care and security. There was plenty of evidence from our visits to care establishments and talks with residents, their relatives and with care staff that this caution, justified or not, is the norm. How then to ensure that residents not only have the opportunity to comment but also feel safe to do so? How to enable people with sensory impairment, communication or learning difficulties to participate fully?

Second, care staff are no more likely than residents to be confident about commenting on current practice and standards. The recent setting up of a support group 'Freedom to Care' for people who speak out about bad practice, testifies to the difficulties and fears of staff in medical, nursing and legal practice. There is no widely established tradition of seeking the views of frontline workers in social care services and the generally low status and morale of residential care workers means that they are even less likely to give their views freely. How might a system ensure that frontline staff too are able to contribute to internal review?

Third, the process would have to address the issues of how to deal with individual views, whether from resident, staff or relative. The difficulty of reconciling idiosyncratic, individual views and preferences with the needs of the care home as a whole are, again, well-known. Nonetheless, if a review is to involve all those with an interest in the home then all contributions have to be taken seriously. How to set up a way of obtaining views which does not lead to false expectations or misrepresentation?

Fourth, the CESSA team was well aware that homes are run by people with their own interests and needs. For owner-proprietors the home is their livelihood: for care managers and staff the home is their work place and they have distinct sets of rights as people and as employees. They are people who have built up experience and knowledge over the years and are strongly identified with the work they do. Their views on the running of the home may not entirely coincide with those of the residents. How may a system of review lead to a fair and reasonable balance between different ideas and interests?

Fifth, there were issues to be taken into account about the value and feasibility of linkage between an in-house system of review and the quality assurance and inspection procedures which are originated outside the home by the encompassing agency and the new arms-length inspection units. How far should the internal process be shaped or influenced by external norms and criteria? The CESSA researchers were well placed to take account of these issues from their development work in registration and inspection.[6]

How the IQA System was Developed

The IQA system was developed in three phases.

First an outline procedure and tools were drawn up using experience from previous research. This was then tried out in a small number of care homes with CESSA consultants taking the lead in setting up the procedures and running the reviews. Initially the focus was on non-elderly client groups. As a result the system was significantly revised and a new set of guidelines and tools produced. In the *second* phase a series of homes used this prototype pack to set up and run a review. Here consultants were fully involved but the managers and staff of the homes took more of a lead. *Finally,* over 100 care homes tried out a revised pack with no consultant support other than a preliminary briefing meeting and the possibility of attending an open forum in their region. In this way the initial ideas of the CESSA team were subjected to practical trial, advice and feedback, not only from managers and staff but also, because of the nature of the system, from residents, their relatives and other outsiders.

Over 130 homes were involved altogether of which the majority were volunteers who responded to invitations to try the IQA pack.

The IQA System

The IQA System is described in a package of materials.[7] This is a free standing 'how to' manual to guide people through a sequence of decisions and activities. It contains a description of the process, a detailed set of guidelines, interviewing schedules and checklists which provide the basic ideas and materials for carrying out a review. People are encouraged to adapt the materials to their own specific needs and to create new tools where necessary.

The first step is to *clarify the purposes and objectives of the home* as the basis of setting clear standards and expectations.

The hub of the review is the *quality group.* IQA advises that representatives of residents, staff, relatives and other external interests constitute the group and that the care home manager or proprietor is neither a member nor takes the chair. The aim is to convene a group that is able to operate in a relatively independent way while utilising both the direct knowledge and experience of *insiders* balanced with the more distanced interest of *outsiders.*

The task of the quality group is to obtain, collate and write up a report on the *views and comments of residents and staff* and, where possible, relatives and other outsiders who have an interest in the home. An outsider member(s) of the quality group interviews residents, staff and relatives.

Confidentiality is an issue and the pack alerts the quality group to the need to address this. If it is important that individuals are not identified the quality group has the responsibility for ensuring that its members respect this.

The pack provides master copies of interview sheets and checklists which are designed to keep the questions focused and simple. The emphasis is on two questions: what is it like to live (work) here? what needs to be different? People are asked to comment on a range of topics which cover, for example, physical care, making choices, and expressing feelings. The quality group is encouraged to revise or add topics to ensure that the focus is relevant to the home and its residents.

IQA advises that the responses are looked at as a collection rather than a series of individual commentaries. This is to discourage placing undue emphasis on the responses of individuals and to encourage an understanding of the general messages coming through, the clusters of concern, the general tenor of the comments.

These ideas are *fed back to the residents and staff* as a means of checking the quality group's understanding of the issues presented in the interviews. This is one way in which the balance between idiosyncratic and more collective views can be discussed. The results of the exercise are then written up in a *report* which should form the basis of *decision-making and action* as well as draw attention to aspects for future review. The pack advises the quality group to plan for the next IQA review and to think about using the document as a way of informing people about the home.

What Is Involved in Using IQA?

The pack contains detailed materials which require careful reading, but homes in the trial phase found it user friendly, readable and clear to follow. The pack appeared successful in describing the essential elements of the process and the majority of the homes in the trial phase completed the review. The pack established not only how to set up a review but also the values and principles on which it is based. For example, most of the homes accepted the importance of involving residents and seeking their views even if they had not managed to achieve this. Equally, the basic value of involving outsiders in the quality group was recognised as an important element in the process.

The time taken to complete the review varied considerably. Obviously the larger the home the more time was required to interview staff and residents but most homes completed in about six months. Some agencies used the opportunity to carry out a more comprehensive review of the purposes and philosophy of their homes, to pool ideas and experience across homes, to promote quality initiatives through training.

There were homes where special measures were needed to enable the residents to comment: these included people with sensory impairment and learning difficulties. Lack of resources or ability to find suitable outsiders to join the quality group also lengthened the process.

What emerged as one of the most important aspects in carrying out an IQA review was the motivation of the home manager or proprietor: without their commitment the review would either not run or become a paper exercise from which no action would flow. Equally important was that someone took a leadership role—not necessarily the head of home or a senior manager—in convening the quality group and supporting the exercise.

The chair of the quality group and the interviewers were those who spent most time on the process although this varied, particularly with the size of the home. The most time-consuming aspects were contacting people to join the quality group, collating and writing up the information from the interviews. Interviewing did not emerge as a major aspect once the people conducting them were clear about their task. The implications for staff time were relatively low: extra meetings and cover for staff on the quality group and some staff meetings to discuss issues arising and action to be pursued. On the whole staff time did not appear to be a significant cost in running an IQA review.

Other resources needed related to duplicating checklists, the administration of the quality group, preparing and publishing a final report. Most homes found these were more of a cost in people's time than in money. One or two homes used a computer to analyse the material from the interviews and found this a valuable way of handling and displaying the information.

The homes which prepared for the review by involving all levels in the home and agency were, on the whole, able to get on with the process and use the comments and views most effectively. Although IQA is an in-house review, back-up from the organisation as a whole is an important element. Many of the items which arise from the interviews have implications for senior management, for budgeting or staffing which can only be addressed at higher levels in the agency.

Equally the understanding and commitment of staff within the home is crucial. Preparation helps people to feel part of the review rather than objects of comment or scrutiny.

How Successful is IQA?

It is significant that about 90 per cent of the homes participating in the trial completed a review. On the evidence of their experience the

IQA system is remarkably successful in enabling residents and frontline staff to comment and contribute to an internal review. The exent to which residents were involved varied but their participation was valued: in many cases staff were surprised at how balanced and helpful residents' comments were. Many homes recognised afterwards that residents could have been more involved if they had been helped to prepare or had more support in expressing their views. However, given the lack of experience or, in many cases, any tradition of seeking residents' views, the IQA system must be seen as a significant step forward in enabling people to comment and participate in review.

On the whole residents were cautious about expressing their views and it is probable that, first time round, people are not prepared to be very open. However, there were clear indications that if the review led to discussion of important issues and some action was taken (even if the matter was not fully resolved) then residents and staff felt that their views were taken seriously and were more confident about speaking out.

Staff in many homes were somewhat doubtful and anxious about the exercise. There were those who feared that residents would be critical or that their own views might be misunderstood. It was important that these kinds of concerns were recognised in the initial stages of the setting-up of the review.

Overall, homes obtained information and comments that were highly valuable and often less critical and less costly than feared. The issues which people wanted addressed were not always those which managers saw as important: there were several cases where the priorities of staff were different from those of the residents. The use of feedback meetings allowed these differences to be discussed.

The results of the IQA review in the trial homes fell into five categories.

—First, people seemed to enjoy the experience even when there were tensions between staff and resident interests or between outsider views and those of staff. On the whole people responded to the opportunity to review the work of the home themselves.

—Second, staff generally gained confidence in their work through being involved in discussions, from giving their views and from the feedback from residents. The feeling was that their work was being valued even where aspects of the way the home was run were being criticised.

—Third, outsiders learned about the home and felt involved. Family and carers were well represented on the quality groups. They expressed pleasure in being involved although many were careful in their comments on the home or were fearful of upsetting the staff.

—Fourth, residents were helped to see that their views were valued. In most of the homes there was an increased sensitivity on the part of staff and managers to the needs and rights of residents and, perhaps of most importance, recognition that residents can speak for themselves and contribute to the way the home is run. There were many examples of direct benefits: in the form of changed practices—like choice of meal times, staff spending more time doing things with, rather than for, residents; in physical improvements—locks on residents' doors, new showers, redecorations.

—Fifth, the IQA process provides a means of reviewing standards and of presenting the work of the home to outsiders. In many cases, home managers and proprietors were keen to demonstrate that they had the means of ensuring quality of service: the IQA emphasis on the involvement of residents was an attractive element in this.

Commentary

The experience of the homes involved in the development of IQA suggests that the system does provide care home managers and proprietors with a comprehensive and workable system for running an in-house review. One of the key findings is that the majority of the homes were successful in including their residents—some to a greater extent than others—in commenting on the way the home is run. This marks an important step forward, particularly since the homes which successfully completed a review included homes for people with learning difficulties and elderly people with dementia—groups which can too easily be labelled 'hard to reach'.

Another step forward is the recognition of the contribution that outsiders can make and this links with the increased awareness of the position of relatives that is being promoted by the newly formed Relatives Association.[8]

Although it may be unlikely that IQA would be used by residents, relatives or staff to make serious complaints there was clear evidence that it helps to generate a climate in which people feel able to complain.

The results of using the IQA system appear significant in the short-term with a good chance of being sustained and built on given appropriate support. One of the features of the success of the trial runs is linked with the setting up of a quality group. This provides a way of organising and supporting the review while at the same time keeping it distinct from day-to-day management. It is probably true, however, that in the longer term the success of in-house reviews will depend on the extent to which higher levels in the organisation accept and respond to the work done by individual establishments.

Establishments certainly valued the opportunity to take the initiative in running an in-house review. Some saw it as a chance to explain what they do and to inform others. The fact that most of the reports produced from the trial runs of IQA included a balance of positive or affirming and critical comments or recommendations for change suggests that internal review has a value in its own right as well as being complementary to external processes of quality assurance or control.

In summary, IQA makes a very positive contribution to helping people—frontline staff, residents, relatives—to speak out. It is successful in good part because it has a clear set of values, it makes sense to staff and managers because it is grounded in good practice and the emphasis on balance—between residents and outsiders, between residents and staff—appeals to people's sense of fairness.

2. WINDOW IN HOMES

Links Between Care Homes and the Community

The Wagner Review made clear the view that residential establishments should be seen as a part of the community in which they are located: 'It should not be necessary to speak in terms of links with the community—residential establishments should so clearly be a part of the community they exist to serve'.[9]

However, evidence to the Review included commentary on the isolation of many care homes and drew attention to the kind of difficulties this can generate. The more cut off the home the more likely it is that residents will not be able to use the full range of services and opportunities available in the locality. The fewer the visitors the more likely it becomes that restrictive regimes and bad care practice will be not be noticed or challenged. On the positive side, the development of links between the home and its local community can help to ensure that residents retain their rights as citizens through, for example, exercising choice, being actively involved in local activities and using community facilities.

As part of the Initiative, the Social Care Association (Education) was commissioned to develop a better understanding of the ways in which care homes and their local communities interact and try out ways of promoting links.

The aims of the programme were:

—to promote more contact between residential establishments and local communities;

—to stimulate more involvement by residents in the life of the home and in outside activity;

—to create more feedback on standards of care.

The Challenge

In looking at the links and relationships between homes and their community, the SCA researchers were asked to tackle a relatively new set of ideas and, as yet, ill-defined aspects of residential care practice and development. There were few, if any, existing frames of reference or previous studies on which the work could be based. Notions of linkage between an institution and its environment may not be new in a theoretical sense but there has been no systematic attempt to examine the particular relationships of care homes. Traditionally they have been seen as places apart, often located away from town centres, cut off from the main social and commercial 'shipping routes' and out of sight.

The dominant model of residential care has been that of an institution providing total care where residents expect to stay throughout their life. The internal world of the residential community has been, in many cases, expected to provide all that was needed for a fulfilled life. This notion has been increasingly challenged, especially by those working for and with people with learning difficulties. The principles of normalisation, for example, have helped to dismantle such models of total care and to replace them with integrated approaches which expect and enable people to use the mainstream services and facilities which are available to all in the community.

The programme was thus dealing with some of the legacies of institutionalisation (in the histories of people and of establishments) and much of the work, therefore, had to be concerned with exploring current thinking and practice and with beginning to define the nature and benefits of links between care homes and their community.

How the Work Was Developed

One of the first tasks was to adopt a working definition of the term 'community'. This was an essential undertaking given the diffuse and variable meanings that are ascribed to community in different policy, practice and theoretical contexts. As the result of a literature review[10] the team took the term to refer to: 'the mix of formal and informal links which make up the network of relationships between the residents who live in an establishment and other people outside'.[11]

The programme identified a number of aspects to explore through practical work. A series of projects were set up, each involving a cluster of care establishments working with a consultant. Care homes and agencies were invited to participate in the work and this generated a lot of interest. It seemed that exploring or developing community links was attractive and about 40 homes worked with the SCA.

Each care home involved was invited to complete an establishment profile: this was a way of gaining a picture of where the home was as a basis for considering community links. Like the IQA review and the Training for Care Staff work this was a way of encouraging and enabling managers and staff to look at the home as a whole and how the project work would help to enhance the quality of life experienced by residents.

The Nature and Purpose of Links

The projects focused on individual care homes across the client groups and care sectors with the aim of learning from current thinking and practice and, in some cases, trying out new approaches. The programme did not develop a single model or approach: the various projects looked at rather different aspects and each was shaped by the interests of the particular homes involved. In order to understand the nature and purpose of links with the community it is helpful to distinguish four broad categories.

A. Residents' Personal Links and Networks

Across CHI, people living in care establishments told us—or implied in what they were saying—that one of their main difficulties was that of isolation. People referred to social and emotional isolation as well as physical constraints on getting out and about.

In terms of the role and tasks of staff, this implies discussion and work with people on an individual basis both to understand and preserve existing contacts and to help people to create networks and make new friends inside and outside the home. This might include, for example, recognising the importance of memories—helping someone to preserve these can be as important as actual contacts. But equally, residents themselves, their families and carers can be active and take responsibility for ensuring that such relationships are established or maintained.

Several projects focused on such aspects:

—facilitating a friends group in an SSD home for elderly people;

—supporting the setting up of a befriending scheme in a voluntary home for people with learning difficulties;

—reviewing admission procedures in an SSD elderly people's home;

—an oral history project with a local school in an SSD home for elderly people;

—looking at ways of involving local people through voluntary and social links in an SSD home for elderly people;

—looking at a scheme for helping formerly homeless men to establish ordinary links.

B. Residents' Use of Mainstream Facilities and Opportunities

The benefit of questioning established patterns of using—or not using—outside facilities was apparent to us across the client groups. Staff and residents easily fall into an acceptance of what is or is not possible which is more often defined by traditional notions of what people want or are able to do than real life aspirations and capabilities. Equally, there are all sorts of ways that people can contribute to the life of the community and have a voice in what is provided and how things are run. These may be very individual arrangements or made for the residents on a more collective basis. Supporting people through the transition from residential care to more independent living means knowing what is available in the community as well as understanding the continuing links that the individual might need with staff and friends in the home.

These possibilities imply outreach work from the home and discussions by staff and by residents with, for example, local clubs and leisure centres, political organisations, campaign groups, day centres, sports facilities, churches, housing associations, colleges, job centres, transport firms, etc.

A number of projects explored such issues:

—recruiting volunteers to extend the range of activities for people with learning difficulties and sensory impairments;

—work on policy around risk-taking as a means for staff to facilitate community links for people with learning difficulties;

—the role of volunteers in enhancing links for people with communication difficulties;

—support for young people leaving care in two SSD children's homes: a large establishment with a specific leaving care unit and a small home providing outreach support for leavers.

C. *The Home as a Whole: Its Relationship with Friends, Neighbours, Outside Bodies and Agencies*

Across CHI, care home managers and proprietors were concerned about the way their establishment was regarded in the wider community. These concern were fuelled in part by anxieties about attracting contracts and customers. In homes for young people and those viewed as deviant in some way the concern was about preserving the rights of and opportunities for the resident and dealing with the stigmatisation and discrimination that care homes and their residents can face from neighbours and the wider community.

Such problems imply a role for leadership: the task of representing the establishment as a whole is one for management but here too, there might be a role for residents and frontline staff.

The home as a whole may be a resource for individuals and groups from the community. There are potential conflicts here between the interests of residents and those who use the home for other reasons but the notion of the care home as a resource centre is well established.

Several projects were involved in exploring such aspects:

—work to promote positive local links for a number of homes with a poor or stigmatised local reputation; these included an establishment for young people and a therapeutic facility for people with drug and alcohol problems where past links with community were seen as a problem;

—helping to build a positive reputation for an elderly people's home following a major incident of malpractice;

—supporting staff of an SSD-run elderly people's home in developing a lunch club to encourage links with local black elderly people in a multi-ethnic inner city community;

—work of a private elderly people's home in providing support services to local elderly people;

—plans for an SSD 'linked service centre' for elderly people;

—plans for reusing resources of an SSD home for people with physical disabilities to cater for other people with disabilities living in the area;

—work on community links as an aid to preventing institutionalism in three voluntary homes for former hospital patients;

—looking at two dispersed residential schemes for people with learning difficulties.

D.   *Internal Relationships*

One of the aspects which SCA researchers considered was that of internal relationships. The culture and climate of an establishment is a reflection of the way people regard and respect each other—as colleagues and as fellow residents. Creating a climate of openness and trust in which people feel that they belong, feel secure and feel free to comment and participate fully is a management responsibility but not management alone. The work of IQA, for example, shows how residents can share in reviewing life and work in the home.

Window in Homes anticipated that good internal relationships might well be the basis for good communication and relationships with outsiders and projects working on these aspects included:

—the roles of volunteers or external workers in supporting residents' committees or self-advocacy groups in two homes for people with learning difficulties;

—the role of voluntary committees in a voluntary home for elderly people;

—enhancing communication within the home, including the use of keyworkers.

Learning from the Projects

The experience of the projects highlighted a number of issues about promoting and maintaining links with the community and these are briefly outlined.

Involving Residents

As with other CHI work, involving residents was a significant issue. Although the aim of the work was to improve residents' quality of life, there were a number of cases where they were not invited to participate. The problem appeared to be that staff were not used to involving or consulting residents: promoting community links took the form of staff thinking about the issues rather than discussing ideas with residents. Where residents were involved the home was able to appreciate their life experience in new ways. As with the IQA review, residents' views revealed differences from those of the staff, their priorities were often different: they wanted less supervision and support than staff thought was necessary; they wanted opportunities to make choices and take risks. It was through advocacy groups and working with outsiders (eg, volunteers) that this kind of information came to light. The projects raised a number of questions about how residents may be supported in making contacts outside the establishment.

The projects showed that thinking about links with the community can help to increase awareness of residents' needs and rights to do ordinary things, to make personal relationships, to do things their way. They also demonstrated the kind of active role residents can take and the responsibilities they can take on.

Using Volunteers

Several projects involved volunteers both full and part time. The most successful projects were those where the volunteers worked directly with residents and helped them to express and carry out their ideas. Developing confidence to speak out, to go out and to make new contacts was a first step for one group of people with learning difficulties. The volunteer was able to work slowly over a period of time. One of the points to emerge was that there are important limitations to what volunteers can achieve—especially if they are involved on a temporary or short term basis. For their work and its benefits to be sustained, the role they fulfil has either to be taken up by the staff or taken on by the residents themselves.

Equally on an individual basis the benefit to the residents is only as good as the volunteers. They need to be available, acceptable and reliable: where personal relationships result the residents can benefit greatly but casual popping in can be confusing and patronising.

Improving Communication within the Home

The work on internal relationships echoed that of the IQA development projects. The climate or atmosphere in the home, the way people relate to and respect each other is indicative of the kind of links that the home has with outsiders. For example, where there are difficulties between staff or a lack of flexibility in the way the home is run, it is less likely that the home will be open and welcoming to others. Work on improving communication within the home is one way to help people to express themselves and understand each other better.

Benefits for the Home as a Whole

The benefits for the home as a whole were explored in relation to improving public awareness and understanding of the home. Many of the homes involved in this programme came to understand more about the importance of the way the home was perceived by others in the community and to see that this was something which they could actively influence. Managers and proprietors, but also care staff, were helped to see the role that they could play in extending relationships and discussions with other groups and interests in the locality. The importance of, for example, talking directly to people in the community, to the press, to neighbours, was highlighted in several projects. Being a good neighbour is about positive, reciprocal relationships not only avoiding criticism and censure.

The Practice Guides

The work has resulted in a series of booklets which aim to offer tried and tested ways of thinking about links between residential establishments and communities which we would encourage others to try. Each focuses on a different aspect of linkage drawing on project experience. These include:[12]

—'Voluntary Links': focusing on the role of volunteers and the relationship between their role and that of staff.

—'Positive Images': which looks at how a care establishment can work to improve its relationship with the local community. This draws on the experience of a childrens' home with a poor public image which staff took active steps to improve.

—'Giving and Taking': a consideration of the role that a care home can play as a resource for individuals and groups from the local community.

—'Communication Begins at Home': this looks at internal communication and suggests that good links with the community are based in good relationships inside the home—between staff and between staff and residents.

—'Lasting Impressions': looks at the way positive links can be established.

Commentary

The work of A Window in Homes has helped to focus attention on the family and social links that residents have inside and outside the care establishment and on the relationships that the home has within the local community. One of the things to be confirmed is that traditional ways of seeing the home as a place apart do limit opportunities for pursuing an ordinary life. The projects showed how easy it was for staff teams to accept the current pattern of things and not to question what other opportunities might be created—for themselves as well as the residents.

It was clear across CHI that there are residents in every home who feel isolated and constrained: this was as true for younger people as the elderly. It was also clear that people need help to reach out and make new contacts. For many there were physical difficulties like transport or being able to communicate easily but what caused even greater isolation was lack of confidence and anxiety about seeking companionship, social and emotional support.

Staff cannot be expected to fulfil all these needs. But A Window in Homes highlights the responsibility of management and staff in creating the kind of climate in which these things can be discussed. The work certainly challenges notions of care. The projects showed that it was often staff who had a difficulty about taking risks: residents were clear about what they wanted to do and the possible consequences.

3. TRAINING FOR CARE WORKERS

The Wagner Review and reports which have followed looked at the link between staff status and morale and the provision of high quality services. The recommendations from these reports and reviews are consistent in suggesting the following set of relationships: low morale is associated with stress and being undervalued as much as with low or anomalous levels of pay and long hours; low morale leads to high rates of sickness and staff turnover and lack of commitment to the work; lack of training, opportunities for staff development or job enhancement contribute to staff feeling undervalued and confirms low status; stress arises from tensions within staff teams which come, in turn, from lack of understanding of the nature of the work and from poor support from management. This analysis links together key elements of ensuring quality service: the recruitment and retention of good staff through the provision of training, staff development and appropriate management support.

The Wagner Review recommended that: 'every establishment should be required to draw up a staff training plan . . . (which) should be subject to inspection procedures'.[13] The National Institute for Social Work (NISW) was asked to develop training approaches and materials for basic level care staff.

The aim of the work was to improve the quality of residential care in both the statutory and independent sectors by promoting basic training of care workers of a kind which could readily be arranged and supervised by the managers of the homes, and which would equip them with essential competencies in line with the National Vocational Qualifications framework. The kind of training to be developed was, therefore, concerned with the provision of locally managed, in-house opportunities.

The Challenge

The work was being conducted at a time of considerable change. The implications of community care implementation are particularly significant for training—especially at senior and middle management levels in statutory and independent sector organisations—

as people were expected to take on new aspects of work and to acquire new skills and knowledge. The agenda for training is being determined by these needs and these fall primarily into such areas as financial management, financial and legal aspects of purchasing and contracting, assessment of services, case management and inspection procedures. In this climate, training for basic level workers in residential care services has not always been seen as a priority.

In personal social services in both voluntary and public sectors there has been little, if any, tradition of developing services through job enhancement and investment in the workforce through career development opportunities. Few agencies have developed an approach to staff recruitment, training and development in a way that integrates these functions with existing and changing operational and practice requirements of the service. A general trend has been for social service department training sections, for example, to allocate time and resources to in-house courses for specific purposes, for example, to respond to new legislation. Seconding people on external courses is relatively expensive and has been seen as something for the individual rather than as a means of accessing knowledge and experience for wider dissemination within the agency.

Training and staff development—as distinct from providing supervision for care workers—has not always been seen as a management responsibility. The development of the national system of vocational training and qualification (NVQ) has pushed managers and senior staff more clearly into the role of trainer albeit in relation to the individual learner.

In contrast, the NISW approach was based in the belief that practice development is an inherent part of service provision and, as such, an essential element in management. Individual and staff team support, training and development, were thus seen as an intrinsic management responsibility and part of an integrated approach to ensuring relevant, effective, good quality services. The challenge to the programme was to demonstrate how care homes could be helped to develop training plans which were consistent with the purposes and objectives of the care home and which would meet the needs of a staff team working together as well as provide individuals with induction and foundation training.

General Principles

The basic principles adopted by the NISW team were:

> —that training opportunities should be based in and consistent with the values, practice principles and purposes of the service and that these should, therefore, be made explicit;

> —staff training and development should be an integral part of service provision and quality assurance and therefore training for care workers should be understood and planned within a broader frame of staff and team development;

> —the process of learning should be integrated with practice: training events and materials should be designed or adapted for each establishment or group in order to ensure that it complements everyday practice: it follows that training needs should be defined by care staff themselves;

> —the importance of developing a climate for learning through enabling care staff to make full use of their existing knowledge and experience and through increasing awareness of the importance of staff training and development;

> —it is consistent with this that managers' competencies in training should be developed as part of their management role.

The programme was therefore as much concerned with the contexts within which learning and developmental opportunities are provided—the organisational climate, training policies and culture, management attitudes—and with the processes of planning and providing training as with the knowledge and skill content and the way these are packaged.[14]

The programme was not only developing appropriate training approaches and materials. It was also seeking to demonstrate the essential connectedness of training and staff development to the wider aspects of care provision and their place in ensuring quality of life for residents.

How the Work Was Developed

The programme adopted an *incremental* approach, building on grassroots assessment of training needs. Projects were led by independent consultants working within an agreed set of values. There was no attempt to design and try out a single training model: projects were encouraged to develop a range of approaches to meet local needs and objectives. The aim was for participant care homes or agencies to build from and adapt the NISW-led projects both 'in-house' and by creating links and networks with other care providers.

Several projects involved groups of homes working together, across sectors and across client groupings, to pool resources or as a means of developing training and operational networks.

The projects were *interventionist* in that they aimed to produce change, but *participative* in that they worked with care managers and workers rather than imposing change on them.

In all, 22 projects were carried out involving over 100 care homes.

A Generalised Account of the NISW Projects

Most of the projects were supported by consultants apppointed by the NISW programme. This is an important aspect to bear in mind since the degree of external help and resource has implications for the general relevance and applicability of the approaches. Although the projects were diverse, they shared basic values which were highly consistent with the overall principles and values of the programme. What follows is a generalised account of the way that the projects were set up and run.

Setting Objectives

Each project set out with clear and explicit objectives. These were negotiated with each participant home or agency while also fulfilling the central purposes of the NISW development programme. In all cases this involved discussion with the home managers and usually staff were also involved. Residents were rarely included at this stage.

Auditing

Most of the projects began by carrying out an appraisal of the current work of the home as a means of identifying gaps or areas of practice that needed to change. This provided the basis of looking at training needs and from this the development of a training plan for the home as a whole. The audit covered a number aspects:

The Purposes and Philosophy of the Home

One of the features of the audit approach was an emphasis on recording the aims, purposes and philosophy of the home. There were several examples where managers and staff discovered that they did not have a clear or shared understanding of what the establishment was setting out to achieve.

Characteristics of the Home, the Residents and the Staff

The audit gathered basic information about the home, about the residents and staff. As well as physical details, the audit recorded indicators of the health of the home in terms of staff turnover, levels of stress, communication difficulties, levels of and type of staff support.

Assessment of Quality and Current Care Practice in the Home

Various questions were included about care standards and practice and how these are reviewed. Many projects used a simple self-evaluation checklist published by NISW as a means of inviting staff and residents to think about and discuss the running of the home.[15] This was the point at which several homes included residents in the process.

An Agenda for Training

An appraisal of the current work of the home was used to develop a profile of the training needed to address some of the issues raised. The final stage of the audit process was to consider what action needed to be taken and, in particular, the kind of training that would help to meet issues revealed through the audit.

Designing and Running the Training Programme

Designing the programme for training involved decisions about the overall shape, size and duration of the training events, the content, the style and level of teaching/learning, about use of existing materials or packages, people to be involved and how it would be reviewed. This included decisions about resources in terms of materials, staff time and cover, management involvement and about who would lead the work. The relative benefits of internal or external trainers was a point of discussion for most projects.

Learning from the Projects

Benefits for Staff

Many care staff had had little in-house or any other form of training. For them the opportunity to talk about their work and learn from others in an unthreatening way was highly valued. People were committed and could see the relevance of the training since they had been involved in deciding what was needed. The general results were an increased awareness of residents' needs and rights and a greater sensitivity to the different needs and perceptions of residents. Staff also developed confidence in themselves and each other. People realised that they had skills and knowledge which they could share with colleagues and that it was possible and rewarding to learn from others. Staff had a better sense of the purpose of the home and there was a marked increase in staff morale.

Benefits for Residents

Benefits for residents were more difficult to assess: few were directly involved in discussing training needs or in the training activities. The impact will come indirectly as a result of changes in staff attitudes and practices and there were clear indications that this was happening. Examples from the homes participating in the development work included: staff being more available; taking time to sit down and talk to residents; doing a cleaning job with a resident rather than when they were out of the way; changing breakfast arrangements to a buffet-bar for flexibility; ensuring that people have privacy when seeing the doctor. These might be seen as small items but they symbolise very significant changes of thinking in some places.

Implications for Management

The initial audit looks at current practice and management. Home managers found it useful to promote thought about what needs to be improved. The exercises provided an opportunity for managers and staff and, indeed in some cases, residents to open up discussion about the home and what it seeks to provide. There were several examples where staff teams were surprised to discover that there were important differences of perception between them about the purposes of the home and about how they could best meet the needs of their residents. These kinds of discussions certainly had management implications not only in developing a relevant and appropriate training plan, but also for day-to-day issues. There were, for example, homes where the process revealed considerable difficulties in staff groups, management problems and resource shortfalls. Here there could be a danger that because the audit was being conducted in the course of looking at training needs that a solution to such difficulties might be sought within a training framework. The experience of the projects certainly emphasises the relevance of the NISW approach in seeing training as an intrinsic part of management responsibility in service provision.

Collaboration between Homes and Agencies

The projects in the research showed that high level collaboration within and between sectors is possible although the most successful examples were those that built on existing networks. Private care consortia and a network of agencies in the mental health field, for example, worked together to provide induction and foundation training for basic grade staff as a way of pooling resources and learning from each other. The benefits of such collaborations were clear in terms of increased staff interest both in their own work and that of other agencies or homes, increased understanding of the needs of a particular user group, and sharing training resources.

The Costs of the Approach

The major input for the projects was management and staff time in discussing and setting up training programmes, attending sessions, and arranging staff cover. Some homes pooled resources with others but here too, they needed plenty of time for joint planning and discussion. However, many of the establishments involved in the projects saw training as an intrinsic part of the general running of the home and could not entirely separate out the cost of this element from day-to-day work. Many homes, for example, used regular staff meetings to address some aspects of a training programme, like residents' rights or ideas about team-building.

Some homes might, on the experience of the projects, need some outside support to set up and run a programme but most were able to carry out some form of audit and set an agenda for a training programme.

Programme Outputs

Most of the projects involved in the Training for Care Workers programme produced reports and material which are of general interest and value. They represent a rich source of experience and information which is practical and relevant although, in many instances, the approaches would need to be adapted to local requirements.[16]

In addition the programme is publishing a distillation of the experience of the developmental work in the form of a comprehensive manual.[17] This guides care home managers and proprietors through the process of assessing their training needs. This draws on the projects' experiences up to the point of designing a programme of training. The manual provides a step-by-step guide through a sequence of tasks and activities:

—building a picture of the current work of the home;

—assessing training needs from this;

—deciding on priorities for training;

—setting aims and objectives;

—designing a programme;

—evaluating the plan.

The approach is broadly the same as that followed in the projects with a great deal of detailed materials to help people through a complex set of tasks. In doing so it covers many of the points of difficulty identified from the projects. Each section includes an explanation of what needs to be done and why, a series of activities to be followed, practical ideas and examples.

One of the issues on which the manual provides clear guidance is that of working out the training implications that arise from an assessment of the home.

The guide includes many references to residents and the benefits of including them in the activities—as a way of understanding their needs and as a means of ensuring that residents' views are heard and valued. The position of the residents is not, however, given prominence in the same way as, for example, the IQA review places residents' interests as central.

Comment

One of the important outcomes of the projects was to show how readily people with very little, if any, training can respond to the opportunity to think about their work and the kind of support that they might need. Although for many the idea of training was somewhat threatening initially, the approach adopted by the consultants and other trainers involved in the research—which was participative, enabling people to learn from each other—quickly overcame such difficulties. Much of the success of projects seemed to stem from people feeling that their ideas were valued and that the work that they were doing was also being valued: the rise in confidence, commitment and morale which flowed from this was very apparent. Equally, people became more receptive to the views of others and this included a greater ability to understand the needs and the experience of residents.

The training approach developed by the NISW research focuses on the relationship between the aims and purposes of the home and a training and staff development programme. It is service-based and involves grassroots appraisal of the kind of training required to help meet those objectives. The work has emphasised the value of local and in-house training opportunities serving the home as a whole rather than courses or qualifications for individuals. Involving staff in setting the agenda for training has led to their greater commitment to and understanding of the work. Team discussions of this sort also helped people to recognise management difficulties. This grounded approach has highlighted the importance of integrating planning and management in a way which includes issues of staff recruitment, training and development.

The shifts in morale and confidence that can result from team based and in-house training demonstrated the potential value of this kind of approach. Some projects did experience difficulties but these were generally about coping with change, recognising and managing the balance between the different needs of staff and of residents.

4. INFORMATION AND CHOICE

The importance of providing information for people seeking and using services was underlined by the Wagner Report. The emphasis which the review placed on the rights of the resident helped to highlight the essential role of information in underpinning real choice for service-users. In the period since then there has been a growing understanding of the importance of information—for management and the internal requirements of service organisations and for service-users. The implementation of community care, with its emphasis on consumer-led services and individual case management, has led to an increasing recognition of the need for up-to-date and comprehensive information about the range and availability of care services in the community. Purchasing and providing agencies are concerned and on two fronts: first, to be able to disseminate accurate information about the services they offer for potential customers and second, to have information about other agencies.

The motivation on both counts may lie either in promoting consumer rights—people have a right to accurate information about services and the alternatives available to them—or in a market-led concern that the agencies' services (products) are known about by potential purchasers.

The Policy Studies Institute (PSI) was commissioned to look at provision of information. Originally this was to address the needs of those either in or considering a move into residential care. With the publication of the White Paper and subsequent legislation on community care, the objectives of the PSI programme were revised to encompass the much wider task of providing information for users of personal social services.

The aim was to produce general guidelines for providing comprehensive information for service-users and their carers. This was a large undertaking for a number of reasons. Information provision and use in the field of care services has not, until very recently, been recognised as an essential element in the internal functioning of service organisations although the setting up of internal systems has been expanding rapidly. In this context, providing information for users embraces a relatively new set of ideas and involves a shift in emphasis and focus on the part of provider agencies.

The project was also a considerable undertaking because of the potentially enormous range of services relevant to different groupings with different needs.

At a later date an additional project was commissioned which focused in more detail on the information needs of people considering or living in residential care homes, although, in the event the work focussed only on elderly people. The booklet 'Home Truths'[18] was developed through discussions with a number of care home managers and proprietors and written with them particularly in mind. It provides guidelines and advice about the kind of information people require when considering entering residential care and the exchange of information needed to ensure that managers, residents and their carers are able to make well informed decisions.

Information for Users of Personal Social Services

The team developed a model for providing information which took SSDs as the lead agency. The decision was based on the views that:

—SSDs have a lead responsibility for community care services (eg, in assessment, care management, purchaser and provider, inspection) and therefore an intrinsic interest in the range and availability of services across the client groups and sectors of provision.

—The Children Act 1989 and NHS and Community Care Act 1990 include a number of requirements that users of services are provided with information, thus placing social service departments in a key position in providing and ensuring that information is available.

—SSDs are the only agency with the potential resource in time, money and influence to set in place the policies, strategic planning, operating procedures, personnel (including inter-agency links and securing the collaboration of other agencies) and technology required.

How the Work Was Developed

Early work by the PSI team involved looking at the *underlying issues*[19] and finding out about the *information needs of service-users* and how they seek information.[20] A survey of written information provided by local authorities and residential care agencies was carried out, analysed and published as *guidance on presentation and information design*.[21]

A Consultative Group, of people with an interest in information provision from 12 local authority SSDs, was set up to provide a forum for discussion, information and practice exchange. The SSDs represented were selected by the PSI researchers as all had made some progress in developing systems for providing user information. They included a range of shire and metropolitan authorities, political characteristics and geographical location.

The kind of developments which they had been pursuing included a system based on a comprehensive audit of services available by client group across the whole authority; a system based on setting up information access points linked to GP surgeries; partial moves towards a collaborative system with user groups; a federation/agency network approach; initial moves to developing an information strategy. The group also included an action researcher concerned with the development of information systems for people with physical disability.

Projects were set up in collaboration with six of the SSDs on the consultative group. The aims and focus of these were decided in two ways. The Consultative Group identified a series of important aspects of information provision which the researchers then explored in practice. Most of these coincided with the interests of particular SSDs who were then able to pursue these with help from the PSI in a series of pilot projects.

The elements of information provision listed by the Consultative Group and covered by the projects was extensive but not necessarily comprehensive. The researchers did not attempt to construct a model of information provision for users or expect the projects to follow a common approach. Each project group worked independently drawing on the experience of the PSI and from other SSDs, learning as the work progressed.

The kind of work undertaken by the pilot projects included information for specific groups or communities like black and ethnic minority groups, information for people with learning difficulties and the provision of information for the elderly about new care management arrangements; producing information for professionals in other agencies and information for front-line staff; other projects considered consultation with users and carers; reaching and meeting the needs of dispersed rural communities; at a strategic level, developing an information policy for providing information to service users; links with the inspection process, providing information about complaints procedures and the role of information in community care planning and consultation.

The projects thus covered a number of very different concerns ranging across geographical, client group, communication, strategic planning and resource considerations. None of the projects set out to integrate these different aspects or to devise and implement a full system. But each was expected to contribute to the overall thinking of the SSD concerned and to act as a catalyst for further development. In this way the PSI acquired practical information from a series of projects which formed the final guidelines.

Learning from the Projects

From the SSDs' point of view, the projects were seen as partial approaches which would help to establish the importance of information provision for service users as well as achieving certain specific outcomes. The projects provided staff with valuable experience in thinking about user information alongside the tasks of community care implementation. The links between service provision and user needs were thus highlighted and so formed the basis—however small—of a more integrated understanding of the need for and purposes of information.

The Validity of Work on Information for Users

The pilot work took place in authorities where the responsibility of the SSD in providing information for users was established in principle. However, the extent to which this work was accepted as having some priority varied considerably. On the whole the projects were operating at the margins of other aspects of SSD work. For example, some were financed because of the necessity of informing the public about complaints procedures. In another, materials were prepared to inform people about the new assessment and care management arrangements—a central operational change—but the work was paid for from a small amount of money available to the information officer.

The general message was that information work was valid but there was a tendency to define it in terms of providing information *about* services of the SSD.

A User Orientation

A few projects were able to explore information needs from the users' point of view.

In one for example a detailed survey was carried out to try to establish the needs of rural or dispersed populations and how the SSD might meet these. Customer services staff carried out a questionnaire survey, interviewed local people and agencies in a number of areas and canvassed the views of SSD personnel in order to obtain a picture of information needs, networks and priorities.

Another project set out to reach a 'hard-to-reach' group—people with learning difficulties. Individuals and user groups were invited to explore the kind of information that people with learning difficulties and their families needed and the different ways of making this available. The project group tried theatre, video and role play techniques, all involving the users themselves. The work was important, not only because it achieved some direct results in terms of information shared and valuable relationships set up, but also because it revealed to those involved the slow and sensitive nature of working in collaboration with user groups.

Apart from these projects there was a marked tendency to see and talk of the service user as a recipient of information about services. The general tenor of the work fell into the category of informing people about the work and services of SSDs. Although people spoke of the information that people need in order to understand alternatives and make choices, the actual plans and work did not maintain this orientation. The issue of taking the users' point of view and consultation with user groups was, however, a strong theme in the two day workshop of the Consultative Group.

Policy Issues

Several projects where the aim was to produce information for the public about SSDs own services found their work hampered by internal lack of clarity about policies, priorities and eligibility for services. One project group took a very considerable amount of time to ensure that the wording on a pamphlet was accurate about the availability of a service, in principle, yet did not imply that all who were eligible could, as a right, obtain that service. The level of anxiety about misrepresentation at a time of reduced levels of service showed clearly how the provision of information to the public can run straight into political issues. SSD personnel were—or felt—unable to inform the public about actual service levels. This group, and others, were able to voice their concern about lack of clarity at the policy level and lack of thought about people's right to information.

An Information Strategy

Although the pilot projects were pursuing different aspects of information provision, all agreed that an essential goal was that the SSD established a policy on information. In some cases SSDs already had an information strategy but these related to *internal information* handling and use. The issues were about the internal needs of the organisation within which, if they featured at all, *user requirements* tended to be located as a marginal aspect of operational or service management. Internal strategies tended to be dominated by technological systems and issues of compatibility rather than specifying the nature and purposes of collecting, disseminating, accessing and using information. It was not surprising, therefore, that progress in the pilot projects towards the formulation of an overall SSD strategy for users was slow.

Recently, however, there is evidence that the implementation of care management systems is highlighting the need for better information across the range of services.

Time Scales

Most of the projects took longer than anticipated. The duration was obviously related to the amount of time that staff could give to the work but the commitment of locals and their seniority also made a difference. One of the most time-consuming activities for staff within the SSD was agreeing the content, style and format of information leaflets and other materials for public distribution.

A significant but not surprising finding, from the project which most successfully involved service users, was the considerable amount of time needed for real consultation, sharing ideas and reflecting on the results with a range of other people.

Costs and Resources

Given the partial nature of the projects, it has not been possible to come up with the costed model for the provision of information. The issue was discussed in the Consultative Group and the experience of the various authorities represented suggested a number of aspects of cost and resource that would have to be borne in mind.

First, there was agreement that the major cost would be that of staffing. Whatever system was adopted it would need dedicated staff and this would mean, depending on the size of the authority, at least the appointment of a full-time information officer with specific responsibility for user information. Second, it was generally felt that since information should be an intrinsic part of service provision the cost of providing suitable materials and keeping front-line staff up-to-date within the organisation at local levels should be costed into general operational budgets. Third, the cost of technology would depend very much on the extent to which the system might be based in computerised data handling. Opinions were somewhat divided about the extent to which information technology could deliver the kind of interactive system which would be necessary since it would require a considerable amount of contact and networking between an information unit located within the social service department and other agencies.

The Guidelines

The guidelines, 'Informing People About Social Services'[22] are published in four parts, each addressed to a different audience and tackling different tasks. They are styled as a package of guidance for SSDs on developing information services for users and the public.

'Part I—Meeting the Need for Information'

Part one is addressed to directors of SSDs and elected members. It sets out the reasons why an information system is needed and why the SSD has responsibility to meet legislative requirements and general needs in this area. The guide emphasises that the public and potential service users have a right to good information in terms of entitlement and knowledge of alternatives. It refers to a general trend towards greater consumer participation and control through initiatives like the Patient's Charter. The guide takes a clear line that the provision of information is for the benefit of potential and actual service users.

'Part II—The User Information Policy'

Part two provides guidelines for policy makers and senior management on the formulation of a comprehensive approach to setting up a system of information provision. The elements of a policy and some of the key features of the system are identified. For example, the guide advocates that management and user information services should be integrated and that the system should serve those who need and use information rather than be determined by the technology.

A section on working with other organisations refers to the need for SSDs to work jointly with and obtain information about other service and information providers. The guide does not emphasise, however, the essential aspects of collating comprehensive information about the services, ie, about direct care services and about information and advice services—provided across the sectors and covering the needs of a wide range of client interests.

'Part III—Developing Information Services for Users'

Part three is a practical guide for those involved in setting up and running a system. The guide advocates that a central information unit and clearing house is established 'to co-ordinate and facilitate information work throughout the department and to liaise with external information providers and other agencies' and that its remit should be authority wide.

The guide refers to the need for appropriate training for information work and the roles of receptionists and frontline staff are identified as of particular importance in responding to people's need for information. The resource implications are discussed in relation to the overall view that everyone in the organisation has a part to play in providing good information and that this should became an integral part of service provision. A section refers to the need to obtain the co-operation of and to work with users, voluntary and private sector agencies, other departments of the local authority, the health authority and national sources of information.

The final section discusses practical aspects of getting the message across: for example, thinking about the needs of different groups, how to reach rural communities and people with special needs, using different means of providing information, designing materials, mapping possible outlets and contacts, using the media.

'Part IV—The Summary of Legislation and Guidance'

The fourth part provides a comprehensive listing of recent legislation and central guidance as these refer to or have implications for information provision.

Commentary

The guidelines are the result of careful consultation with over 12 LA SSDs and are a comprehensive synthesis of current ideas about what constitutes good practice. Inevitably some of the aspects—particularly those relating to user participation and consultation and collaboration between the SSDs and other agencies—are described in ideal terms since thinking here has outstripped practice. The guides represent an important step in promoting strategic thinking about the information needs of service users and do address some of the concerns that any SSD would have in tackling such complex tasks.

The queries that can be raised relate to the role of the SSD which the guidelines promote. During the programme's work the emphasis on the SSD as the lead agency remained but the nature of the task described in the guidelines is one which requires a high degree of collaboration with outside agencies and key information sources including the participation of service users. We can note some of the issues which might make it difficult for the SSD to collect and make information available on a comprehensive basis. One of the key questions is whether a SSD can make the cultural shifts necessary—first to distinguish between internal, management requirements and user-focused information needs, second to open up boundaries between internal operations and functions, and third to set up collaborative working links with a variety of outside agencies including user organisations.

The scale of the shifts needed should not be underestimated. Across the CHI there were numerous examples where staff were anxious about releasing information to outsiders and occasions when information was shared with fellow professionals (and outside researchers) but not the residents concerned. The climate of caution was especially clear in inspection units. Understandably inspection officers are feeling their way in a new environment and many units have not worked out their policy on how to handle reports which are expected to be available to the public. The picture adds up to one where we should expect it to take authorities some time, first to recognise the responsibility in information provision, to clarify the task and embrace a user orientation and then to move into a new kind of relationship with service, information and advice agencies.

The fundamental query, however, relates to the kind of information which the public and potential service users require and the level at which it can be effectively collated and disseminated. The experience of specialist, voluntary organisations which work at a local level, like Age Concern and MIND (and also the growing experience of professionals involved in assessment as part of care management) shows the detailed and local nature of the information needed to provide individualised and integrated services. An issue which client groups and user organisations can address, in some measure, which a central SSD-led system is unlikely to do, is that of providing the kind of qualitative information which people seek when deciding between service alternatives. The experience of the federations involved in the National Disability Information Project set up by the Department of Health to improve information services for people with disabilities will be important here. They will help to show how far information needs to be targeted towards special interest groups, collated at a very local level, and how far it is possible to provide such information through collective or multi-agency systems.

The Caring in Homes Initiative and Positive Answers

In summary we can ask in what ways the Initiative contributes 'positive answers' to the issues raised by the Wagner Review. The results of the work—in the form of guidelines and practice manuals—have, in most cases, only become available very recently. We will have to wait to see how relevant and useful they are when taken up by a wider public. Meanwhile, the experience of the homes and agencies who were involved in the research demonstrates a number of positive ideas and trends to come from the Initiative.

Arguably the most important is the contribution that the CHI programmes have made to understanding more about the way that residents themselves can be involved. The experience of the projects has shown that people are able to make a lively and thoughtful contribution to the running of the home and, that where criticisms are made, these are fair and balanced.

The experience of CHI is also important in demonstrating some of the ways in which opportunities can be created to enable people to speak out. These have included helping people to contribute to a process like an IQA review, being part of an advocacy or other user group, and generally being encouraged by a shift in attitude or climate in the home to one that is more open and friendly.

Another important aspect of the CHI work is in showing the value of frontline staff being more involved in reviewing and thinking about the way a home is run. The more staff had the opportunity to share ideas and learn from each other, either in a process of review or in training sessions, the more sense of purpose they developed, a greater sense of working as a team and, as a result, felt more valued and committed to the job.

An interesting aspect of CHI has been the opportunity to look at care practice and management across the client groupings and to understand what quality of life means for different people. Writing and thinking about residential care services has tended to be dominated by provision for the elderly: the CHI experience shows that there is much to be learnt by looking at practice and care management across the care groups.

A final observation concerns the generally positive outlook which care home managers and proprietors have in spite of the considerable upheaval which residential care services and community care generally have been going through. Although people were anxious and concerned about the future, about funding, about contracting and registration criteria, there was an underlying and strong feeling that it was residents who mattered most. The idea that residents should and can comment on standards of care and express their own views about lifestyle and opportunities was widely accepted: even where people were not sure how to put such ideas into practice, this was seen as the positive way forward.

Notes

1. Wagner, G., (Chair) *Residential Care: A Positive Choice. Report of the Independent Review of Residential Care*, 1988, London, HMSO.
2. Youll, P. J. and McCourt-Perring, C. A., *Taking the Initiative: Changing Practices in Residential Care* (provisional title), 1993 (forthcoming).
3. Wagner, 1988, op. cit.
4. Kellaher, L., Peace, S., and Willcocks, D., *Living in Homes: A Consumer View of Old People's Homes*, 1985, BASE in Association with CESSA.
5. Willcocks, D., Peace, S., and Kellaher, L., *Private Lives in Public Places*, 1986, London, Tavistock.
6. Peace, S., and Kellaher, L., *Making Sense of Inspection*, 1990, London, HMSO.
7. CESSA/PNL, *Inside Quality Assurance*, 1992, PNL.
8. See Chapter Nine, 'Wagnerian Reverberations'.
9. Wagner, 1988, op. cit.
10. Elkan, R., and Kelly, D., *A Window in Homes: Links Between Residential Care Homes and the Community. A Literature Review*, 1991, London, SCA.
11. Freeman, K., and Kelly, D., *Communication Begins at Home*, 1992a, London, SCA (Education); Freeman, K., and Kelly, D., *Voluntary Links*, 1992b, London, SCA (Education); Freeman, K., and Kelly, D., *Widening Horizons*, 1992c, London, SCA (Education; Freeman, K., and Kelly, D., *Giving and Taking*, 1992d, London, SCA (Education); Freeman, K., and Kelly, D., *Positive Images*, 1992e, London, SCA (Education); Freeman, K., and Kelly, D., *Lasting Impressions*, 1992f, London, SCA (Education).
12. Freeman, K., and Kelly, D., 1992a, 1992b, 1992c, 1992d, 1992e, 1992f, op. cit.
13. Wagner, 1988, op. cit.
14. Douglas, R., and Payne, C., *Organising for Learning. Staff Development Strategies for Residential and Day Services Work: A Theoretical and Practical Guide*, 1988, London, NISW.
15. NISW, 'Self-Evaluation Chart', *Care Weekly*.
16. See for example: Daley, T., Miller, T., and Wood, K., *Introduction to Care Planning*, 1992, London, NISW; Mabon, G., *An Induction Programme*, 1991, London, NISW.
17. Hillyard-Parker, H., Mabon, G., Payne, C., Philipson, J., and Riley, M., *How to Manage Your Training: Developing a Training Plan* 1993 (forthcoming), London, NEC/NISW.

18. Dawson, C., Bloch, A., and Moore, N., *Home Truths*, 1992, PSI.
19. Steele, J., *Information about Residential Care: The Underlying Issues*, Information Policy Working Paper 1, 1990, PSI.
20. Roberts, S., Steele, J., and Moore, N., *Finding Out About Residential Care. Results of a Survey of Users*, 1990, PSI.
21. Lewis, D., *An Information Design Audit of Information About Residential Care*, 1990, PSI.
22. Steele, J., Hinkley, P., Rowlands, I., and Moore, N., *Informing People About Social Services*, 1993, PSI.

CHAPTER NINE

Wagnerian Reverberations

It is not an exaggeration to state that the Wagner Report—and the developmental work immediately engendered by the basic principles it enunciated—constituted something of a watershed, in terms of residential care in particular, and social care in general. This chapter presents brief accounts of some of the initiatives currently in hand. But these are only an indication of where current trends could lead. The philosophy promulgated by the Wagner Report is now accepted—at all levels, and over all sectors. 'Positive Answers' indeed, which could result in a positive future, despite (as ever) the inevitable constraints in terms of finance.

Complaints Procedures in Residential and Nursing Homes: Encouraging the Right to Say

Introduction

The subject of complaints is much discussed, but often little understood by those who most need to know about it—service providers and users. The NHS and Community Care Act 1990 has introduced a requirement for local social services authorities to have formal complaints procedures. Such procedures are regarded as an essential safeguard of users' rights to have their say. Where local authorities contract for services with independent providers, they are likely to expect such providers to have their own complaints procedures, and to show how these will be made to work.

The Registered Homes Act 1984 requires care homes to inform residents about how they can make complaints. The Wagner Report stressed the importance of residents being able to exercise control over their own lives, including having the 'right to say'. The requirement for authorities and homes to have a procedure for complaints is increasingly seen as meaning more than a paper exercise in which the channels for complaint are described. The Department of Health and the Scottish Office have both issued Guidance which shows that the success of complaints procedures depends not only on a clear and easily understood procedure, but also on a climate of communication which encourages users to feel that they can express their views, and which encourages staff and managers to respond appropriately. In other words, the success of a *complaints procedure* will depend on the *complaints process*, through which such procedures will really be made to work.

Making Complaints Work

The word 'complaints' can generate negative feelings in providers and staff. Residents may be reluctant to express their views, for fear of reprisal or through reluctance to cause trouble. Considerable cultural change is needed in many homes to make complaints procedures work successfully and become part of an essential process of communication and feedback within a home.

There must be a formal procedure, understood and 'owned' by everyone involved. This is the safeguard which ensures that when things go wrong, there are proper channels for resolving the problem. But this process will only work if it is operated in a climate of openness where listening to the user is the central value. Neither the formal procedure nor the climate of 'listening' is sufficient on its own. Each feeds the other.

Successful complaining should be:

—easy;

—fruitful;

—taken seriously and responded to quickly;

—acknowledged by those living and working in the home as a positive element of feedback aimed at improving the quality of life of the resident;

—an important focus of the home's training.

However, it may not always be able to satisfy the complainant.

There are incentives for everyone in making complaints work. In particular:

—**Residents** will be encouraged to develop autonomy and independence, to know that they will be listened to and that they will be central in the running of the home.

—**Staff** will develop greater responsiveness to residents, gain in confidence, and increase job satisfaction.

—**Providers** will satisfy their residents, improve the quality of their service, satisfy the registration authority and develop their market share.

—**Inspectors** will be provided with more effective means of monitoring and handling complaints.

The Wagner Development Group's last piece of work was to ask a Sub-Group to look at ways of translating the theory of effective complaints procedures into reality in homes. It sought to dispel the negative reactions, and to promote the necessary culture change. Listening and responding sensitively to users were its central values.

The Sub-Group saw little point in seeking to develop model complaints procedures, since homes already have them, but persuaded the Department of Health to fund a project to produce a package of video, audio and written materials which could improve the climate for complaints through training and by raising awareness in homes. The package is now in preparation by LBTC: Training for Care, under the guidance of an advisory panel drawn from the Wagner Development Group, and will comprise:

Video Tape

This will provide a brief introduction followed by a series of linked but separable vignettes or cameos illustrating good or bad ways of handling complaints in homes, for example:

—a complaint about food;

—a complaint through a relative of rough treatment at bathtime;

—a complaint by one resident against another;

—a complaint not made, although its cause is clear.

The vignettes will emphasise the importance of recognising the individuality of residents and each person's unique needs and point of view. They will be situations which will 'ring a bell' amongst a wide range of viewers, helping them to think about and recognise common themes, and leading to awareness of the importance of good communication in complaints procedures. In addition to the 'subject' matter of complaints, themes illustrated will include:

—dealing with 'difficult' behaviour; and with the habitual moaner;

—issues arising from uses of forms of restraint;

—consideration of special cultural or religious needs;

—different approaches for different client groups;

—the user's right to say, balanced with the rights and responsibilities of everyone living and working in a communal setting.

Audio Tape

To parallel and supplement the video tape, useable independently of the video where such facilities are not available, and for people with visual impairment, with similar material and themes to those of the video.

Written Materials

A series of work cards/work books related to the vignettes or cameos in the tapes, but taking users into more depth concerning, for example:

—the legal position on complaints in homes;

—the role of complaining in ensuring the quality of life in homes;

—complaints as an element of communication in the home;

—complaints and the home's value system;

—the importance of the individual in all aspects of running the home;

—the management role in resolving complaints.

Further information is available from Peter Riches LBTC: Training for Care, 9 Tavistock Place, London WC1—Tel: 071 388 2041.

The Relatives Association: Seeing Homes in the Round

There was one group of people involved in residential care who did not take part in the deliberations of the Wagner Committee. These were the relatives of those in homes. There were indeed references in the reports and papers to the importance of relatives, friends and local communities; but the work was focusing on the residents, and the possibility that relatives might have their own perspective, and views about their own contribution, was not taken into account.

Ten to 12 years ago, except for the few who could afford to go to private nursing homes, most people thought of hospitals as the place they would eventually be moved to when they could no longer be looked after at home or in a local authority residential home. As the elderly population explosion mounted, the hospital services began to respond by modernising wards and making them more homely, but this was not sufficient and the situation was met by the great increase in private residential care and nursing homes.

Initially the relatives saw themselves as visitors. They were used to being visitors to hospital wards, to being allowed to visit at only certain times, and to accepting the professionalism of the staff. They might observe but could not question. Their situation in relation to homes was a difficult one. They had accepted, or had decided, that care in a home was the best course for the elderly person. They could often see that the care being provided was not as good or as individual as they would like it to be. They were often racked with guilt because for one reason or another they could not provide the care themselves.

They could see how difficult it was for the staff of the home and they felt it would be unreasonable to complain—sometimes because they were afraid of the consequences for the resident if they did so. They could no longer identify with 'carers' who were looking after their elderly people at home, sometimes throughout the day and night. They felt they could not go to carers' groups and talk about their problems. They were often very isolated and seldom met others in the same position. Some homes had established relatives' groups, mostly to help with fund-raising and outings, but most relatives felt themselves to be on the outside; some preferred this, but for many it was a great strain.

At the end of February 1992 a group of relatives who found they had all experienced similar problems founded the Relatives Association for the relatives and friends of older people in homes. The Association met a felt need and within a year it has succeeded in creating a general awareness that the role of relatives has to be better understood and worked out jointly. If elderly people are *not* to be 'put away' into homes it is important that their relatives should be able to do what they can to help with their care, and be their allies in maintaining their individuality. Of course relatives can be awkward; they can fade away; there can be ill-will within families. But very many are deeply concerned.

The Association at present offers an advice service, over the phone and by correspondence, to people who want to talk over their feelings—often of bereavement or guilt—about the elderly person being in the home, and discuss any problems they may have with the home, or ask about practical and financial questions. The Association's aim is to help callers take things up with the homes themselves; but sometimes, if asked, they may mediate on behalf of the relative.

There are now complaints procedures, but many relatives see these as very much a last resort. They do not want to have to complain: they want to work with homes. The Association is therefore working with relatives and homes to help promote relationships within homes in which it really is possible for relatives individually and collectively to play as full a part as they can in contributing to the running of the home.

As numbers grow, the Association hopes that networks of relatives will develop within each local authority area, able to support each other and to feed views into the advisory and planning structures and be consulted by them.

The Relatives Association will also have a keen interest in future joint studies on the lines developed by the Wagner Committee, into the delivery of good quality care. They can see the crucial importance of staffing, and the problems that surround this. They are interested in cost/quality factors. They are interested in developments which may bring homes more into local communities, both for the advantages and disadvantages which these bring to existing residents. Above all, they have a keen personal interest in the future. Many of these relatives, the children of the very elderly people in homes, are now themselves in their late 60s and 70s. They see care in homes very much as a personal matter which they view through the eyes of their own very elderly relatives, and through their own eyes as maybe future residents.

The Relatives Association is an Association for the relatives and friends of older people in homes. There are other similar associations: for the relatives of those with a mental illness who are in long-stay hospitals or homes—'MARCH'; and for relatives of those with learning difficulties/mental handicap—'RESCARE'.

All the Associations recognise they have a difficult role. Relatives must not take over from nor presume always to know what is best for the individual resident, but when residents have difficulty in making their views known, many relatives feel an obligation and deep need to try to ensure that they are understood. Not only do residents need their families as allies, the families have their need for understanding too. Relatives can offer a great deal to the individuality of life for the resident which homes might not be able to afford to provide.

The development of mutual understanding among all concerned is the prime aim of all these Associations.

Further information is available from: The Relatives Association c/o Counsel and Care, Twyman House, 16, Bonny Street, London NW1 9PG—Tel: 071 284 2541 or 081 201 9153. MARCH, Woodtown House, Alverdiscott Road, Bideford, N. Devon. EX39 4PP.— Tel: 0237 470889. RESCARE, Rayner House, 23 Higher Hillgate, Stockport. SK1 3ER.—Tel: 061 474 7323.

Counsel and Care: The Right to Take Risks

In 1992 and 1993, Counsel and Care contributed to a series of conferences throughout the UK on the issue of the right to take risks for older people in homes. This conference season was made possible by a grant from the Mental Health Foundation following the publication of the discussion document 'What If They Hurt Themselves'. This document, the discussion and seminar which preceded it, and the conference programme are all part of Counsel and Care's continuing work on the quality of care for older people in homes.

The conclusions of 'What If They Hurt Themselves' made it clear that there was a need for guidance on the issue of risk-taking and restraint. Such guidance is needed in relation to individual residents, good practice for staff, policies for homes, guidelines from local authorities and principles spelt out by the Department of Health.

The conferences and links with others involved in this work provide an ideal vehicle for Counsel and Care to work to produce model documents to meet the needs outlined above. The widest possible consultation with all those interested and involved is essential. The drafts that follow, which are extracted from Counsel and Care's subsequent publication called 'The Right To Take Risks', need such help if they are to be meaningfully enhanced.

Principles of Care Relating to Risk-Taking by Older People in Homes

1. Life is full of risks. Many people feel that risk-taking adds a sparkle to their lives. Without risks, life would be impoverished. Normal life is about responsible risk-taking and risk assessment.

2. The elderly residents of residential care and nursing homes should have as far as possible the same rights as people living in their own homes. Their legal rights as individuals are not affected by admission to a home.

3. Restraining someone without their consent is unlawful. It is not permissible to assume consent where it has not been expressly given.

4. There is a difference in law between intervening before and intervening during an event. Intervening before a resident has embarked on what a staff member may consider to be an inappropriate activity and in order to prevent them hurting themselves is not permissible without their consent. Intervening appropriately, for example by discussing the implications or holding an arm but without exerting force in an activity which is already in progress and is proving to be dangerous and thus discouraging the resident from continuing, is in accordance with the duty of care. Allegations of assault are more likely to arise from preventive action taken before an activity begins, and of neglect if no action is taken or if action is taken too late.

5. Restraining residents on the instructions of third parties is not acceptable. Unless residents come within the scope of mental health legislation, no other person has in law taken on responsibility for them. If advocates or proxies take decisions for residents, there must be recorded agreement for this to happen.

6. A thorough care plan should be agreed for each resident on admission and frequently reviewed thereafter. The plan should include all details of risk-taking agreements so that resident, relatives and staff are all in possession of full knowledge and their expectations of each other are realistic.

7. A resident must be party to any agreements about their own care plan, as their express consent is required for any subsequent action to be lawful.

8. Confused residents seldom have absolutely no moments of lucidity. Such moments may become less frequent as time passes, but staff and relatives who know the resident well and spend time regularly with them will be able to harness those moments to gain an understanding of the resident's own wishes as and when the opportunities arise. Discussion with residents to ascertain their views must be attempted, though it will not be possible to plan in advance the meetings when this can happen. Staff need training in order for them to become competent to spot and interpret residents' wishes from their behaviour rather than their spoken words. The starting point is that residents are trying to find some way of communicating their wishes rather than the assumption that they cannot. Assumptions should not be made about a resident's competence in one area of activity because of a seeming lack of competence in another.

9. The use of any restraint should be contemplated only as a last resort after exhausting all other options. It must be agreed and recorded in the care plan, in accordance with procedures laid down for that establishment. It should be time-limited and speedily reviewed.

10. Medication should never be used to control behaviour or as a punishment nor without the consent of the resident.

11. The objective must always be to provide the least restrictive life style to residents compatible with reasonable care and safety and at the same time to offer opportunities for stimulation and fulfilment similar to those enjoyed by older people outside homes.

Considering Risk-Taking for Each Resident

1. Ensure that prospective residents and their relatives have adequate information about the home and what it offers when considering admission. Risk-taking and restraint should be specifically mentioned. No home should be expected to offer a totally safe environment.

2. Discuss and agree expectations on both sides so that everyone is clear on the realistic limitations and the potential for disagreement about this subject in the future is diminished.

3. Before admission or very soon after, set in place a detailed and agreed individual care plan to which all involved are party—the

resident, their relatives and other carers, the staff, the GP, the resident's advocate or agreed proxy if there is one, and other involved individuals and professionals. This must include statements about agreed levels of risk and how decisions are to be taken on these on a day-to-day basis.

4. Gather information about the resident and with due respect to privacy make sure it is available to appropriate staff. This should include details of the resident's life in the past and aspirations for the future as well as their views on how they are to be cared for.

5. Ensure that the care plan is regularly reviewed, that alterations are clearly recorded, and that all concerned agree to any changes.

6. Recognise that changes in residents' care plans may allow for more and not less risk-taking in the future. Do not assume that risk-taking has to diminish with length of stay or increasing age.

7. Make arrangements for regular discussions about the care plan with the resident, their relatives, staff and other relevant people.

8. Ensure that the care plan is regularly referred to by care staff and is a working document, not just something which is completed and filed away.

How to Deal With Restraint and Risk-Taking in Care Plans

1. Individual care plans should be completed for each resident.

2. The plan should address all aspects of care for the individual. This should therefore include risk-taking.

3. The care plan should be agreed by everyone who has an interest in the resident's care: the resident, their relatives and other carers, staff, the GP, the resident's advocate or agreed proxy, and other involved individuals and professionals.

4. Point 5 is a checklist of headings related specifically to risk-taking and restraint for inclusion in the care plan. It is not comprehensive. Under each heading detailed discussion is needed to determine the way in which the home will undertake to attempt to meet the resident's own wishes about their lifestyle.

5. The headings under which risk-taking and restraint need to be addressed should include:

   —privacy and use of rooms and bedroom,

—going out alone;

—visitors;

—visiting outside the home;

—attendance at clubs and centres;

—going to church or other activities;

—engaging in recreational and leisure pursuits;

—carrying identification;

—medication;

—consulting a doctor or other specialists;

—diet and food issues;

—preparing food;

—using kettles and other appliances;

—clothes and laundry;

—financial matters;

—pattern of the day;

—any agreed use of restraint;

—any agreed restriction on choice of activities;

6. For each heading the care plan should show:

   —How able is the resident?

   —What problems does he or she have?

   —What are the aims of care?

   —How are these aims to be achieved?

7. There should be dates and signatures to the care plan and agreement about regular reviews which should also be fully recorded and signed. The information should be easily accessible to staff and to the resident. Beyond those involved in drawing it up and then subsequently caring for the resident, the information in the care plan should be treated as confidential.

8. Decisions about risks are a balance between the right to choice and the resident's competence. The role of the home's staff is to

seek ways to enhance competence, or to compensate for it, or to offer extra support in order to make it possible for the resident to undertake an activity with an acceptable degree of risk.

9. Risk assessment can easily come to rely more on professionals' and relatives' views than the resident's aspirations. To avoid this imbalance, consider the checklist below:

   —identify the risk in discussion with all involved in the care plan;

   —list the advantages, gains and benefits from undertaking the risk, eg increased self-esteem, retention of independence, value of taking own decisions, a wider circle of acquaintances;

   —list disadvantages, losses and possible harms from undertaking the risk, eg physical danger, possibility of attack, getting lost or failure could cause loss of self-esteem, relatives becoming anxious;

   —discount any gains and losses which would in any case occur whether or not the activity were undertaken;

   —weigh the gains and losses according to their level of harmfulness—any harm which is life threatening will be important to consider (eg heavy traffic on a busy road) but any which is insignificant will be less so (eg losing a small amount of money);

   —decide on the likelihood of each gain or loss to see if it is unlikely to happen, may happen, or is very likely to happen

A better decision can thus be taken about how to plan the activity safely or why it is essential to restrict it. It may be that the resident is being unduly protected from an extremely unlikely occurrence, unduly protected from a likely but not dangerous occurrence, or needs additional staff help to undertake the activity in an acceptably safe fashion.

Brief Bibliography

'What If They Hurt Themselves', a discussion document on the uses and abuses of restraint in residential care and nursing homes for older people, 1992.

'The Right To Take Risks', model policies, guidance to staff and training material on restraint and risk taking in residential care and nursing homes for older people, 1993.

Both publications are available, price £5 each, from Counsel and Care, Twyman House, 16 Bonny Street, London NW1 9PG—Tel. 071 485 1550.

Black and in Care: The Bibini Centre for Young People

'Bibini' is an Ashanti word meaning 'black'. It encompasses the aspirations of the Manchester Black and In Care Group who are developing a centre for the support of black young people.

The Bibini Centre stands for:

—self determination;

—valuing cultural diversity and difference;

—challenging racism;

—building on the strengths of black people;

—keeping links, not breaking them;

—young people's rights;

—challenging the discrimination of black young disabled people;

—supporting black young lesbians and gay men.

The Bibini Centre for young people will provide a range of services to support black young people. The Centre is being developed in such a way as to best promote and protect the rights of young people as they have defined them, based on many months of discussion and consultation with young people, carers, parents, workers and local authorities. The work on the project is currently at the stage of determining the financial base for the Centre and it is planned that it will be up and running in 1993.

1. Background

The experience of being 'in care' for many black children is one that negates, denies or undervalues the importance of cultural heritage. It is often an experience, however unintentional, that leaves black children isolated and alienated from their parent communities. This results not only in the loss of a feeling of belonging but also the loss of language, traditions, religion, family folklore, values etc, which are all losses that a black child experiences in addition to the losses associated with coming into care. Furthermore, caring agencies have failed to acknowledge or deal with the effects of racism on black children who in the majority of cases have had to grow up without positive black role models to redress negative views of black people. In this country it is very difficult to grow up feeling good about being black unless you are cared for by people who also feel good about being black. While some young people claim that this did not create problems of identity for them, the accounts of many young people are deeply saddening and the consequences far reaching and profound. Reports of children scrubbing their skin with vim are not uncommon but you do not have to have knowledge of such extreme denial to realise how serious the problems are. For many black children growing up in isolation it is more usual, but no less serious, to attempt to 'sink into the wall', blend in, however you can, minimise the differences, dis-associate yourself from any culture other than English. This has a very damaging effect, distorting self-image and reducing self-esteem.

The Manchester Black and In Care Group (hereafter referred to as the BIC group) was formed in 1987.

The group was set up to:

1. provide a service for young black people in care and ex-care;

2. create a forum to allow young black people to meet and exchange views and opinions, regarding their placement in care;

3. to provide an advisory service which identifies and supports the needs of young black people in care or ex-care;

4. to ensure that all young people in care and ex-care are given equal opportunities regarding race, culture and creed, and in addition, help the statutory/voluntary services to minimise racial discrimination;

5. to educate the public on all aspects concerning young black people in care and ex-care.

The aims are promoted through a range of activities which are carried out by a core group of five workers with the support of an advisory group which comprises young people, carers, members of the community and professionals.

While the work of the group has been valuable, we have only been able to support a relatively small number of young people and despite our campaigning activities, mainstream services to black children remain inadequate and inappropriate. In the years that the group has been operating we have seen little, if any, sign of real improvement and, on the contrary, have witnessed a growing abuse of the group itself. This is evident in the type of work we are asked to take on. Some examples of this are: the request to provide black role models for a black child who the agency intends to place with white foster parents; to provide 'identity counselling' to black children who are living in rural areas where they are the only black people in the family, neighbourhood and school. Practices such as these are widespread and highlight a number of issues:

—that racism in social work practice is a serious threat to the well being of black children;

—that there is a lack of understanding and knowledge about what racial and cultural identity is all about;

—that black voluntary groups are not only open to exploitation but can become a part of the 'problem'—in this case the BIC group is used to prop up bad practice;

—that there is a need for a more concerted and constructive approach.

In the light of these issues, the Manchester BIC group, in consultation with all its members, carers and workers has decided to provide a positive model in caring for black young people.

With the implementation of the Children Act and the work of the Wagner Development Group, the opportunity is here for the BIC group to make a major contribution to improvements in care for black children.

The Manchester BIC group proposes to establish a Centre which will provide a range of services to young people including residential care—the Bibini Centre for Young People. It will be based in premises in central Manchester and will provide the following services:

—**Prevention**—working together with young people and their families to resolve problems, where possible within the context of the family. This work will draw upon the resources that exist within the Centre, within the family and within the community. It may, for example, be appropriate to provide young people with time out through respite care as a means of keeping children and families together.

—**Residential care**—the Centre will provide a 'home from home' for up to ten children between the ages of 10 and 18 (two of the places will be specifically for respite care). The home will be a positive choice for adolescents (14–17 years) who do not wish to live in a foster family or who are unable to live within a family. Except in exceptional circumstances children in the younger age range (10–14 years) will be looked after with a view to their placement with either their own family or with a foster family.

—**Returning to live within a family**—the Centre will work closely with young people for whom the plan is for them to return to live within a family, either their own or a foster family.

In addition to work with young people workers will also recruit, train and support foster carers from the black community.

—**Becoming independent**—assisting black young people who wish to live independently. This will involve teaching appropriate skills, help in obtaining accommodation, help in developing support networks in the community and after-care support.

—**Support to black young people in care and ex-care**—this will provide a base for the 'normal' activities of BIC. These activities will include support groups, advice counselling, and outreach work.

—**Resource library**—the Centre will set up and maintain a resource library for use by young people, carers and workers.

—**Befriending**—it is planned to establish a befriending scheme for black young people who are isolated in residential care.

—**Training and consultancy**—the Centre will offer training and consultancy to local authorities on a range of issues including appropriate care of black children, recruitment of black foster parents, anti-racist practice.

The Bibini Centre will be fully accessible and available to young people with disabilities. It will provide an environment in which children who are 'looked after' have the same rights to 'good care' as children living at home.

Children will be cared for in an holistic sense; this is an approach that not only recognises and seeks to care for the 'whole' child but also places the child within the context of their family and their community. This approach is rooted in the history of black people and encompasses an agreement of needs based on the acknowledgement, understanding and experience of racism and its effects.

This philosophy will underpin the work of the Centre and is essential to ensuring that cultural, religious, linguistic and racial needs are integrated into the overall care of a child.

2. Long Term Plans

The BIC group views the setting up of a Centre as part of a developmental plan which will improve services to black young people across the board. Other services will be based on a constant evaluation of our work and the needs of young people. Future work already identified includes services for young people who are described as having 'psychiatric' problems and other work already underway will provide help to young people in the community who have been or are at risk of abuse. We shall look closely at the needs of the young people within the Centre so that we can identify, for example, reasons why children need care or whether children of a particular ethnic origin are referred more often.

3. Links with Other Agencies

The BIC group values the contribution of many residential workers and it is our plan to develop mutually supportive relationships with other homes in order that we can learn from each other, share skills and expertise and avoid being set up in 'competition' with each other. Likewise we would hope to utilise the expertise of existing black foster parents and workers and complement the valuable work they are doing.

We will build on our networks within the community so that young people gain the full benefit of the riches that exist within the black churches, mosques, temples and community centres.

The Centre will also liaise closely with statutory and voluntary organisations, in particular agencies dealing with health, education and housing.

Where possible families will be fully involved in the personal care of their children. Their views and opinions will be sought as a matter of course. Residential workers will need to have the skills for working with a range of parents some of whom will be supportive and others who may be hostile and obstructive. The principle of working in partnership with parents will be one of the key principles of the home. This will be a crucial element in rehabilitation work, making respite care positive for child and parent and in the recruitment and support of foster parents.

4. Financial Arrangements

The Manchester Black and In Care Group shall seek legal status and recognition as a registered charity. The charity will be established to secure on a long-term basis the welfare and interests of black children in care in Manchester and the North West region. Trustees will be appointed to ensure compliance with the aims, objectives and constitution and to administer funding. The children's home will be an independent voluntary home set up within the Bibini Centre.

While providing good quality care, giving resources and choices to black young people will be the primary aim of the Centre. It will also encompass a range of business activities that will be used to generate income for other developments. An example would be developing positive racial and cultural identity through youth exchange trips and links with African, Asian and Caribbean countries.

Further information is available from the Manchester Black and In Care Group c/o The Black Resource Centre, Old Library Building, Cheetham Hill Road, Manchester M8 7JN—Tel: 061 740 7575.

Residential Work with Children and Young People: A Charter For Children

The Wagner Report was concerned with residential services for people of all ages and many needs. Nevertheless its major focus was on care of adults. After the Report was published there was continuing demand for further work to be done in the interests of children and young peope in residential settings.

This work has been carried out by a multi-disciplinary group chaired by Barbara Kahan and largely funded by the Department of Health. The group has been organised and supported in its work by

Daphne Statham. Members have been drawn from education, social services and health interests, voluntary organisations and therapeutic communities, former young people in care and observers from government departments, education, social services and social work in England, Wales, Scotland and Northern Ireland.

The project has two aims:

—to produce an equivalent of 'Home Life' for children, identifying good practice and providing a useful tool for managers and practitioners, for staff development and for users and their families;

—to provide a resource for whoever might in the future restructure 'Home Life' which would ensure that the specific needs of children would be taken into account and that any revised publication would benefit from the principles which underpinned the Wagner Review of Residential Care.

It was agreed not to restrict the project to residential settings in social services (ie children's homes) but to include boarding schools (omitted from the Wagner Review but highlighted in their Report), health settings and others in which children and young people spend time living in groups away from home. Children and young people in all these settings have some common needs, and that 'Bridges Over Troubled Waters' (published by the Health Advisory Service in 1986) had already demonstrated the need for greater uniformity of practice in various residential services.

The work of the Group has taken place during a period of unprecedented activity and concern with child care issues, and with residential care in particular. Resulting from the review of child care law the Children Bill was drafted and became the focus of extensive debate and consultation. It received Royal Assent in November 1989 (becoming the Children Act 1989). The Act was implemented on 16 October 1989. Between Royal Assent and implementation, many volumes of Guidance and Regulations, as well as other supporting material, was drafted, consulted on and published. The aim of these volumes was to promote and support good practice, and to provide for a minimum standard of care in the settings with which it was concerned. The Children Act 1989 is a major piece of legislation. In drawing together a wide range of legal provision and, in stressing the wholeness of a child's personality and characteristics, it has given a clear signal towards a more unified approach to children's needs, wherever they may be cared for away from home.

A publication is expected by the late spring 1993. It will include legal and historical background material, and a review of the recent and most important national reports relating to residential child care. Examination of the common core of practice will focus on the needs of children and young people in residential settings; their rights, education and health; detailed practice issues; the physical environment; child protection; care and control problems; and management and staff issues including selection and supervision. Specific settings will then be discussed—boarding schools, children's homes, special boarding schools, therapeutic communities and medical and health settings.

The publication will target audiences of residential staff, teachers, nurses, managers of children's homes and special boarding schools, councillors, school governors and policy-makers in local and central government. It will be practical in its approach and the material has benefited from extensive discussion by the multi-disciplinary membership of the group. The group has had valuable assistance in the final drafting from Mark Davies, formerly secretary to the Warner Committee.

Further information is available from Daphne Statham, National Institute for Social Work, 5, Tavistock Place, London, WC1H 9SS—Tel: 071 387 9681.

Charter for Children Steering Group

Ewan Anderson
Durham University

David Berridge
National Children's Bureau

Louise Bessant
Action in Child Care Project

Brian Bishop
Peper Harow Foundation

Ben Brown
Action in Child Care Project

Mark Davies
Department of Health

Joyce Eyeington
Rye Hill Family Care Centre

Dr Bob Jezzard
Guy's Hospital

Barbara Kahan
(CHAIR)

Paul Knight
National Children's Bureau

Dr Marion Miles
Paddington Hospital

Dudley Roach
Social Care Association

Richard Rollison
Mulberry Bush School Central Council for Education and Training in Social Work

John Rowlands
Social Services Inspectorate

Alex Saddington
National Association of Young People in Care

Joan Sadler
Boarding Schools representative

Sister Consolata Smythe
Good Shepherd Centre

Daphne Statham
National Institute for Social Work

Jane Tunstill
National Council for Voluntary Child Care Organisations

Past members

Ratna Dutt
Racial Equality Unit

Michael Hurley
National Association for Young People In Care

Sylvia Miller
Residential Social Worker and former user of Social Services

Observers

Derek Brushett
Welsh Office

Brian Fitzgerald
Department of Education and Science

Denis O'Brien
Northern Ireland Social Services Inspectorate

Wendy Rose
Department of Health

John Smith
Social Work Services Group

Peter Stone
Department of Health

Chris Walker
Northern Ireland Social Services Inspectorate (replaced by Denis O'Brien)

Corresponding Members

Stephen Campbell
Association of County Councils

Deirdre Dowie
Convention of Scottish Local Authorities

Spencer Millham
Dartington Social Research Unit

Chris Payne
National Institute for Social Work

Peter Westland
Association of Metropolitan Authorities

Printed in the United Kingdom for HMSO
Dd296503 C50 4/93 G531 10170